BEAUTY BEGINS AT FORTY

BEAUTY

BEGINS

AT

FORTY

HOW TO LOOK YOUR BEST FOR A LIFETIME

BARBARA COFFEY

ILLUSTRATIONS BY DURELL GODFREY

HOLT, RINEHART AND WINSTON NEW YORK

Published by Holt, Rinehart and Winston,
383 Madison Avenue, New York, New York 10017.

Published simultaneously in Canada by Holt, Rinehart
and Winston of Canada, Limited.

Library of Congress Cataloging in Publication Data
Coffey, Barbara.
Beauty begins at forty.
Includes index.
1. Beauty, Personal.   2. Middle-aged women—
Health and hygiene.   I. Title.
RA778.C67 1984   646.7′042   83-18355
ISBN 0-03-063817-8

First Edition

Designer: Iris Weinstein
Printed in the United States of America
1 3 5 7 9 10 8 6 4 2

ISBN 0-03-063817-8

CONTENTS

ACKNOWLEDGMENTS

My thanks to the following experts who generously gave their time and supplied so much enthusiasm for this project:

DR. MARY BOULTON

RALPH DAMIANO

DR. GERALD IMBER

DR. ELLIOT JACOBS

DR. STEPHEN BRILL KURTIN

JANE KIRBY

PABLO MANZONI

DR. LILA NACHTIGALL

BOB PRESTIANNI

DR. IRWIN SMIGEL

BEAUTY

BEGINS

AT

FORTY

INTRODUCTION

When I was sixteen, anyone past thirty was middle aged. When I was twenty-nine, I wondered how I had gotten there so fast. How could this possibly have happened to me! Then I decided to reassess my values. Maybe *forty* was middle aged.

I remember my fortieth birthday well. I did not feel old at all. I wasn't. Forty isn't old, but somehow it has become a watershed age, mostly for women. At fifty, a man is in his prime. Big corporations promote him to high places. Society considers him an attractive, desirable commodity. At forty, a woman traditionally begins a downhill slide that becomes steeper and more precipitous as she ages. Right? Wrong!

That's the way it used to be. No more. Today, as a woman approaches forty, and for years afterward, she embarks on a fresh new life. If she has been the traditional wife and mother, no longer is the empty-nest syndrome her automatic fate. Once her children are grown, the new eighties woman can start living out a new role. She can enter the work force, joining the millions of women already there. If she is already in the work force, she can look forward to reaching new highs in her career, just as her male counterpart has always been able to do. Or, if there are no economic pressures and she chooses, she can simply sit back and enjoy the fact that, for the first time in her life, she does not have a list of responsibilities as long as an apron string. At last, she can do what she wants with her life.

If you are forty, or approaching it, and do not have a sense of new beginnings stirring somewhere inside you, you are missing one of the most exciting experiences of midlife.

After all, you don't feel old, do you? A recent study by Caldwell Davis Partners, a New York advertising agency, revealed that, on the average, women feel about seven years younger than they actually are. This included women from their twenties to their sixties. Men felt only six years younger on the average! The peak period for feeling good for both men and women was the period between forty and fifty. The one hitch was that men seemed to be able to carry this youthful feeling well into their fifties while women had more trouble doing this. As attitudes continue to change, more and more women will be able to retain this youthful feeling long into their lives.

Midlife *is* an exciting time. If you are not convinced, just look around you. Talk to women your own age and older. Ask them what they are experiencing. Leading pollster Daniel Yankelovich did just this in one study that showed that the thinking of older women seems to have undergone a profound change. More than ever before, women at midlife are reporting contentment with their lives at a time when their mothers—and even their older sisters—used to report feelings of depression and lack of fulfillment. Many of these women are working women who say that whether or not they have economic pressures to work, they *want* to work. Work gives them a new sense of self, a valuable new identity. Even those women who do not work seem to gain satisfaction from the successes of those who do. Women identify with and get vicarious satisfaction from the successes of other women. This has become such a basic truth that advertisers realize it and play on it to sell products. A leading fragrance maker tested several commercials on selected women to see which ones they responded to best. One commercial showed a tired housewife chucking it all at the end of the day and putting on something pretty— including some fragrance—for her husband. A second commercial focused on a working woman who had an equally tiring day at the office. At the end of her day, she loosens up her workday clothes—unbuttons her shirt a button, adds a bright scarf and some perfume— to make herself more feminine. Overwhelmingly, women who saw the commercials identified with the working woman, her new freedom and successes.

At forty or so, most of a woman's traditional family responsibilities are behind her. Ahead is not depression, menopause, and wrinkles. Instead, you have an entire new life to look forward to, years of looking good, feeling good, being ready to achieve the goals you set. In a sense, you are like the envied career military man, policeman, or fireman who puts in twenty years or so, retires at full pension in his prime, and can start a brand-new career. Your "pension" is the wisdom and insight you have gained over the past twenty years. You, too, have put in your time and now you are ready for something new and exciting.

At forty and beyond, most of us have much more going for us than we realize. We tend to think we have never carried a few extra pounds before or we forget the pimples of adolescence or the oily hair that drove us crazy. We tend to gloss over the problems of youth and remember ourselves as slim, smooth skinned, and eternally happy. The problems we have now are all because we are getting older. Nonsense. If you want to clear your head of such notions in a hurry, go into any store where there is a communal dressing room. No matter what shape you are in, I guarantee that you will see worse, and on twenty- and thirty-year-olds. Youth has fat thighs, bumps and bulges, pimples, oily hair, and the blahs. Youth has as much need to hide behind a flattering dress and some well-chosen makeup as middle age does. The big difference between the two is that you, at forty, are wiser. You are also more realistic. Unreachable dreams don't drive you from the peaks of a high to the valleys and beyond of a low. You have a better sense of yourself and what you can do. And what you *can* do now is motivate yourself to look better, maybe better than you have ever looked before. It's possible!

There is a support system waiting to help you enjoy these exciting years. Take a walk through the cosmetic department of any big department store. Crowding the lipsticks and the blushers are a whole new group of products for you. Skin-care products that work while you sleep, while you play, while you sun, while you do almost anything, anywhere. Some are truly little miracles. Look in the Yellow Pages and you will find dozens of exercise salons geared to helping you keep your present good shape or work toward achieving a better one. Look at the labels of the foods on your supermarket shelf. Most of them now tell you how many calories the food contains, how much sodium, how much of certain vitamins and minerals. The support is there. All you have to do is determine what will work for you, and that is where this book can help. It can be your first step toward becoming a better-looking, more fulfilled woman. From this book you can learn how your figure is most likely to change in the next years, and what you can— and can't—do about it. You'll learn about the most flattering hair and makeup for *you*. You'll discover how you can get help deciding whether cosmetic surgery is for you. And maybe most important, this book can help you prepare for one of the most profound but needlessly feared changes, menopause. This book can, I know, stir you to new beginnings, new energy, new faith in yourself and your future. It can make you look at your coming years with the same sense of equanimity my friend Sarah has. She told me this enlightening story about herself.

Sarah had something wrong with her foot. She went from doctor to doctor and spent a small fortune on X rays and special shoes and did foot exercises until she felt she could peel off her toes. She was discouraged. She felt she would never walk without pain again and cursed herself for getting older and "falling apart," as she put it to friends. Finally, Sarah found the right doctor and he found the problem. After a series of treatments, Sarah's foot began to improve. The new doctor made Sarah an orthotic device out of a substance that looked and acted like silly putty. The stuff hardened and molded to the shape of her toes and looked, Sarah thought, like a set of soft, pink false teeth. Reluctantly, she slid the device onto her foot every day and dreaded the time when she would need to buy new shoes. The salesman, she feared, would think she was an old lady.

Time went by and Sarah stopped worrying about her foot so much and even learned to accept—almost—the "teeth" she wore inside her shoe. One day, she was having lunch with a friend who was a good ten years her junior. The friend, whom she had not seen in six months, was limping and sporting a bandage that wrapped around her ankle and disappeared into a sneaker. Her friend apologized for wearing sneakers, explaining that she had been having a prolonged problem with her foot. "My doctor says six more weeks of this and I can take the bandage off," she explained, "but he says I'll just have to adjust to having a little discomfort in my foot whenever I walk or stand a lot." "Don't you feel terrible about that?" Sarah blurted out. "No," she said. "It's just something I'll have to get used to. It's a good excuse not to wear those silly high heels ever again." Sarah, too, had been avoiding high heels for months, because she was afraid they would aggravate the problem in her foot. She felt that not wearing high heels was just another sign of her decline into old age and "sensible" shoes. She thought about the difference between her and her friend's attitude toward a similar problem. Even though her problem was solved and she had no pain, she had allowed herself to be mired down in feeling old. The same kind of problem left a younger woman feeling glad to have an excuse not to wear something she disliked. Physically, Sarah was better off. Emotionally, she was not.

Midlife should not be a time to let every little thing that happens to you make you feel old. It should be a time of excitement, adventure, and pleasure. It should . . . and can be.

CHAPTER 1

IS IT TURNING FORTY OR MENOPAUSE YOU FEAR?

You might think a chapter on menopause is out of place in a book that is mostly about beauty and fitness, even one that is meant for the forty-and-over woman. Actually, I think it is the most important chapter. Women do not usually have trouble turning forty. It is not this age per se that is the problem. What they really fear when they approach forty is oncoming menopause. At age forty, most women feel menopause is just around the corner, and that once they turn that corner, it is good-bye, good looks; good-bye, sexuality; good-bye, femininity. Until you get over feeling that menopause is an end rather than a new beginning, you will not get the most from midlife. Menopause *is* a new beginning, a new freedom. It is a reward after years of family responsibilities. Like any reward, it is not free. There *are* problematic aspects to menopause, but the problems are not nearly as fearsome as most women think. The best way I know to convince you of all this is to talk about menopause right up front by presenting you with facts, not fantasies or myths. This way you will know what to expect. You can stop worrying and begin to enjoy the anticipation of a whole new era in your life. Herewith, the facts.

Betty was thirty-five when she began to notice that her periods were irregular. "I couldn't be having menopause already," she told herself. At forty-four, Helen was sure two missed periods meant she had begun menopause. At fifty-one, Evelyn said, "I'm going to menstruate forever. I'm not going to have a menopause." Actually, all these women were of an age when menopause could occur, but none had actually begun. Betty had her last period when she was forty-nine. Helen menstruated for the last time at fifty. Evelyn was fifty-three when she had her last period. What they all had in common was a dread of going through menopause.

Why, at the first sign of a skipped or irregular period, does any woman past thirty-five assume she is having menopause? Why do women so dread this perfectly natural occurrence? "I think," Betty said, "because we've been made to believe that, in a way, it is the end of your life. It's the end of your sexuality and attractiveness." Intellectually, we may know this is rubbish, but emotionally, it is difficult for many women to believe they can still be attractive, sexually active, and desirable after menopause.

Menopause is, after all, only the stopping of the menses. You don't have your period anymore. How many women do you know who would shed tears at not having a period every month? Who thinks the discomfort and annoyance of bleeding for several days a month is such a high? Then why are we so fearful of the end of it? It is true that you can't become pregnant anymore, but the average woman has no desire to become pregnant again long before she begins to go through menopause. What we fear is the loss of our gender, and it is a damaging fear. If you are still too young for menopause, you are wasting time worrying about it. If you are approaching menopause, you can make your problems worse by worrying.

Take heart from a recent study done by Bernice Neugarten, a sociologist at the University of Chicago, in which women from age twenty-one to age sixty-five were questioned about their attitudes on menopause. Women under thirty held many more negative views than older women who had already gone through menopause. When presented with the statement, "Just about every woman is depressed about the change of life," younger women felt it was more true than the older ones, who *knew* it wasn't true. Forty-eight percent of the young women agreed with the statement, but only 28 percent of the older women agreed! The statement, "Women lose their minds during menopause," elicited the same kind of response. More young women tended to believe it was true than did older women.

The same study showed a striking difference in attitudes about sex. Younger women found it hard to imagine older women maintaining an interest in sex. Only 8 percent of the under-thirty women felt "Women would like to have a fling at this time in life." Thirty-three percent of the thirty-one-to-forty-four-year-old women agreed, and 32 percent of those between forty-five and fifty-five agreed. Only 14 percent of the younger women thought that menopausal and postmenopausal women would be more interested in sex than they were when they were younger, while over a third of the older women felt that sex was more interesting now.

Responses to "After the change of life a woman feels freer to do things for herself" brought out the same differences in attitude between younger and older women. Only 16 percent of the younger women agreed with this statement, while 74 percent of the older women agreed with it!

This study makes it clear that women who have already gone through menopause find it much less fearful than do those who look forward to it. This should be enormously reassuring. Menopause, like most things in life we fear, is not nearly so bad as we think. True, you cannot be a femme fatale at sixty, but would you want to be? Chances are, you will be content as an attractive, well-adjusted woman with lots of good years ahead.

Women, in general, are much more concerned about the physical symptoms of menopause than about a vaguely defined loss of sexuality. Mention menopause, and the average woman still thinks of hot flashes, lack of vigor, palpitations, dizziness, and a host of other symptoms. Most women do suffer some physical problems during menopause, but they are usually not debilitating—unless you allow them to be.

In addition to fearing physical effects, many women fear that menopause means the end of good looks. It is not unusual for a woman to feel that her hair will begin to fall out, her skin will sag, and her weight will balloon. I intend to deal with all of this in the following chapters, but for now, be reassured that this is not the case. Everyone experiences some hair loss with aging, and men as well as women show signs of facial and body sagging with age. But this is a gradual process and there is much you can do to counteract the effects of aging. As for your weight, that is completely up to you. You can retain your figure if you want. In fact, there are many things you can do to make this rite of passage easier and better for yourself.

FIND A GOOD GYNECOLOGIST—AN ABSOLUTE MUST

My gynecologist was one of the nicest men I've known. He was warm, kind, eternally understanding. He always had time for my questions and I never had to sit for long in his waiting room. He listened to my fears and pumped up my courage, especially after my divorce. Through all those years, I sometimes wondered if he would still be around when I went through menopause. He won't be.

He retired ten years early, because he said he could not afford to practice medicine the way he felt it should be practiced—keeping his fees reasonable and booking few enough patients to spend time with them while paying soaring malpractice insurance fees—and he didn't want to practice any other way. I was desperate to find a doctor to replace him. I went through a half dozen referrals, rejecting them all for one reason or another until I finally found someone I felt I could stick with until I passed through the next phase of my life.

If you don't have a gynecologist you truly feel comfortable with, give yourself a fortieth birthday present and find one. You are going to need him or her. If you can find a female gynecologist, by all means use her, but there are not enough women doctors to go around, so my advice is to concentrate on finding the *right* doctor and forget about gender. Finding the best gynecologist for this time in your life may mean giving up the doctor who delivered your children. Often the best obstetricians are not the best doctors to go through menopause with. They can be so geared to the pace of pregnancy and pregnant women that they cannot slow down enough to help you through this life change. Some OB-GYN doctors have little regard for anything but obstetric cases. In addition to being more lucrative, an obstetric case moves along at a predictable pace with predictable results—a baby. Menopause often gives a doctor very little that is concrete to treat. Solace and understanding are not the stock and trade of all physicians. There are a few simple questions you can ask yourself about your present doctor that will help you decide whether you have the right one or if you should start looking for someone new.

HOW TO FIND A GOOD GYNECOLOGIST

Do you regularly have to wait more than fifteen or twenty minutes to see him or her?

If you do, he or she is overbooking patients. Any doctor falls behind schedule once in a while. It is a sign of flexibility. But a doctor who habitually makes you wait twenty or thirty minutes is overbooking. This is the doctor who pushes patients in and out with an assembly-line mentality. He or she isn't the one who will take time with you when you need it.

Do you have to wait for long in the examining room before your doctor appears?

I have sat for what seemed an eternity in chilly examining rooms, my bare bottom poking out of a rumpled gown, pressing against an icy examining table. Finally his highness appears, proffers a few words, then dashes out again. Twenty minutes later, he returns and this time gets on with a hurried examination. He pronounces me "fine" and leaves. I then have to scurry around to find the nurse and exert myself to claim a few more minutes of the doctor's time to ask some questions. If this is a familiar scenario for you, you have the wrong doctor.

Does he or she take you seriously?

This may sound like a profoundly dumb question. It is not. Too many doctors dismiss your fears and apprehensions and tell you not to worry. Too many women have walked around with something really wrong with them because their doctors didn't take the time to talk with them, to listen to a complaint and decide whether it might be related to a serious problem. Those funny headaches, the passing soreness in your breasts may indeed be things that need watching or they may be nothing. But you need to know why a doctor is not worried so you can relax, too.

Does he or she do more than give you a pelvic exam?

A good gynecologist is, for many women, a primary-care physician. You go to him or her for most of your general complaints. If he or she is a good gynecologist, he or she will always take your blood pressure and examine your rectum as well as your vagina. He or she will weigh you and always examine your breasts. He or she will give you an annual pap smear, probably take a urine specimen, and question you a bit about your general health. If your doctor doesn't do most of these things, you have the wrong doctor.

Is he or she associated with a good hospital?

As with any doctor, you want to be certain your gynecologist is associated with a good hospital. Should you have any problems requiring hospitalization, you want to feel confident of the hospital where you will be admitted. If you don't know what hospital your doctor is associated with, ask.

WHAT SYMPTOMS WILL I EXPERIENCE?

One of the most difficult things about menopause is that it is different for almost every woman who goes through it. Another difficulty is that little research has been done on it. Typically, the mostly male medical establishment has not considered menopause interesting or worthy enough to merit substantial research. There are a cluster of symptoms associated with menopause: hot flashes, fatigue, nervousness, sweating, headaches, sleeplessness, depression, irritability, palpitations, pins and needles in extremities, breathlessness, impatience. Many women experience only a few of these symptoms, some experience none, and some many. Unfortunately, there is no reliable way to predict which symptoms, if any, you will experience. The examples of a few typical women will help you understand the range of possibilities.

Janet was forty-eight when she noticed that her periods were becoming scantier and lasting fewer days. Eventually the time between periods stretched out until she was having a period only every four months or so. She found this disturbing because she always felt she might be pregnant. Frequent trips to her doctor reassured her that she wasn't. When she had gone six months with no period, her doctor told her she could assume she was not pregnant nor would she be likely to become pregnant now. He did caution her to continue to use birth control for a year after her last period.

Stephanie, forty-six, noticed that her periods were getting heavier and lasting longer. Once she bled for almost three weeks. Her doctor put her in the hospital for a D and C (dilation and curettage) to be certain there was no problem behind her prolonged bleeding. There wasn't. At this point, Stephanie began experiencing hot flashes almost daily. They occurred at regular intervals, sometimes three or four an hour. She was also tired a great deal and found she slept more than usual.

Linda, forty-nine, menstruated regularly, then abruptly stopped for nine months. She too checked with her doctor to be certain that she was not pregnant. During the nine months without periods, her breasts were tender almost continually, and off and on she had a heavy, clear, thick discharge that she found annoying. She, too, had hot flashes and noticed that when she had the discharge, the hot flashes reappeared. All during this time, she found that she felt unusually irritable. After nine months, she started menstruating again and did so regularly for another six months. Then, abruptly, she stopped again, this time for good.

Though all three of these women experienced different symptoms at different times during their menopause, they are all pretty typical of what you can expect. Most women experience hot flashes at some time during their menopause. For most women, the flashes last only a minute or two and are confined to the upper half of the body. They come and go over a period of several years. Many women seem to notice flashes more at night or in the early morning. Some doctors call severe hot flashes experienced at night "night sweats," and they can make sleep difficult.

Nervousness and irritability are almost as common as hot flashes. Many women become aware that little things bother them more than they used to. One woman reports "yelling at my husband for leaving his glasses next to the bed, for crunching his breakfast cereal too loudly, for doing almost anything at all." Another woman, a supervisor in a large office, found she lost patience easily with the women who worked for her. Feeling teary is another common complaint. "I would burst into tears over a broken nail or a broken glass, stupid little things." Women often say they are not necessarily depressed, they just cannot seem to control their tears.

During this period of your life, it is important to remember that your symptoms are real. Doctors used to dismiss menopausal symptoms as "all in your head." We are now learning, thanks to some new research, that these symptoms are very real. Menopause causes profound changes in a woman's body. For years, your body has been used to having a specific amount of the potent hormone estrogen. At menopause, your body must begin to adjust to less and less estrogen. It is interesting to note, however, that from about age twenty-five on, most women's estrogen levels begin to drop off. The change is gradual, but it intensifies during midlife and there is no denying that the familiar, comfortable body you have lived in for some forty years begins to behave differently. This can be frightening. Just remember that menopausal symptoms are temporary. On the average, most women experience some symptoms—usually off and on—that last from three to five years. They *will* stop; and most women say they feel a new surge of energy, a new interest in life as these symptoms pass—the "new beginning" that we talked about earlier in this book.

WHAT KIND OF HELP CAN I GET?

At the beginning of this chapter, I pointed out how important it was to have a *good gynecologist* during this period of your life. His or her help can be invaluable. Vivian, a forty-six-year-old woman who was experiencing menopausal symptoms, learned this the hard way. Vivian had not menstruated for six months and was suffering from hot flashes. A teacher, she felt terribly embarrassed because she would blush and turn red in front of her high school class. She went to her gynecologist and told him of her problem and asked what she could do. He gave her a short, stern lecture about having to put up with it all and said she should come back in a year or so. Vivian was devastated. Not only had she been denied treatment, but her discomfort had been trivialized. Even if Vivian's doctor felt that estrogen was dangerous in her case, he could have helped by being more understanding. Telling her not to return for a year meant he clearly did not want to hear about her complaints—until they were over!

Unfortunately, there are no magic pills you can pop to cure your symptoms. *Estrogen therapy* is a possibility, but it is not right for everyone and, though it usually relieves hot flashes quickly, it is not clear that it alleviates other symptoms. There is a discussion of estrogen therapy at the end of this chapter.

You will want to *see your gynecologist* frequently during this period of your life. Sometimes, just hearing that other women have experienced what you are going through can help a great deal. Knowing that your symptoms are not caused by any serious physical condition will also help. Hot flashes are the symptoms that send most women to their doctors. If they are serious enough, your doctor may prescribe a short course of estrogen-replacement therapy, though some doctors simply won't consider it. If your life is truly being upset by hot flashes, you should consider seeing several doctors to get a range of opinions. Then you must weigh their advice and decide whether the benefits are worth the risk in your case.

Some doctors believe that *vitamin E* helps hot flashes. Gynecologists I have spoken to say about a third of their patients are helped. Sometimes, just taking something helps because you feel you are doing something positive. Most doctors feel it is safe to take two 400 IU capsules of vitamin E daily, one in the morning and one at bedtime. If you find this doesn't help, you might discuss increasing the dose with your doctor. Stress of any kind makes hot flashes worse, so you should also deal with any stressful situation as directly as possible.

One option that is open to every woman with hot flashes is learning to *dress differently*. There's nothing worse than being swathed in wool and suffering a hot flash. As long as you are experiencing hot flashes, avoid turtlenecks, mohair sweaters, cashmere, anything very warm. *Try dressing in layers*. A suit with a silk bouse is a good idea. A dress with a jacket is another idea, or try a cardigan sweater over a silk blouse. Be certain that whatever you wear under your top layer is presentable. If you work in an office, suits are probably your best bet. You can always slip the jacket off to reveal a pretty blouse underneath. Though synthetics are practical most of the time, don't wear them now. Synthetic fabrics don't breathe and they will stick to you when you are hot and flushed and make you feel even more uncomfortable. Any natural fiber, cotton, silk, linen, even lightweight wool is more comfortable. If you are worried about stains under your arms, go to the dime store and buy shields. They can be pinned or sewn in the sleeve of any dress or blouse. It is also a good idea to toss away your sexy nylon nighty. Most women find hot flashes are worse at night and a nylon nighty just traps the sweat. Find some pretty cotton ones to wear now.

Fear of pregnancy during this time of missed and irregular periods can make you extremely anxious. One thing you can do is *be especially responsible about contracep-*

tion. Don't assume that because you are forty-nine or because you have missed three periods you need not worry about pregnancy. Women have been known to become pregnant in their fifties! You should also *buy a supply of home-pregnancy-test kits* to use when you feel anxious. They are remarkably accurate and can save you a lot of expensive visits to your doctor. They are not, however, foolproof. If you have missed two periods and have any symptoms of pregnancy, do see your doctor.

Joyce, forty-four, was going through menopause. She had all the classic symptoms—hot flashes, irregular periods, and frequent bouts of irritability. She had missed two periods and assumed that menopause was the cause. During the second month, she began to feel slightly "off." Her stomach felt upset in the mornings, she had frequent indigestion, and she noticed she had gained a couple of pounds. Still, she thought nothing of it. Three months later, she still had no period and had gained a noticeable amount of weight, which she couldn't seem to lose. "I can't be pregnant," she kept saying to friends who suggested the possibility. Finally, Joyce became fearful she had a tumor and she went to see her doctor. He looked at her incredulously after examining her and said, "Good lord, woman, you're five months pregnant." Joyce felt she had very few options except to have the baby and hope that all would be well. She had a battery of tests to determine whether there were any problems. The tests were all normal, but Joyce did not have an easy pregnancy. She worried through the remaining four months that something would go wrong. Fortunately, she had a healthy little boy who was a welcome addition to her family, but all such stories don't end so happily.

Doris, forty-five, was married only three years and had

no children. She believed she was going through menopause and was vaguely unhappy that she would never be able to have a child. When she missed two periods, she attributed it to menopause and did nothing. When she started to feel peculiar from time to time, she still did nothing. She felt suspended between hoping she was pregnant and knowing she wasn't, between feeling it would be mad to have a child at her age and wanting very much to have one. Finally, her body told her clearly that she must be pregnant and she went to her doctor. He confirmed her suspicions and told her that at her age, she was taking a great risk having a child. Still unwilling to sort our her feelings and her ambivalence about having this child, she drifted on through more months of pregnancy. She did not have any tests to determine whether or not hers was a normal pregnancy and delivered a severely retarded baby.

Both Doris and Joyce failed to deal with reality. The facts of life during your menopausal years can sometimes be trying, but denying them will not help. It is essential that you *keep in touch with your gynecologist to confirm or deny any suspicions you may have about pregnancy.* Pretending you are not pregnant or being careless about protecting yourself from an unwanted pregnancy are sheer madness.

SEX AND MENOPAUSE

Since many women fear the loss of their sexuality during menopause, it is essential to continue, in fact to enrich, your sex life now. If you fear that you will no longer be attractive or that you will not be able to have sex, you are dead wrong. Many women are at their physical peak from forty to fifty, and even though it is true that you may not be young and gorgeous at fifty or more, you have the same capacity for warmth, giving, gentleness, and sensuality that you have always had. These qualities are exactly those that make the sex act special.

Probably the most important thing to remember is that the large majority of women have an *increased* interest in sex after menopause. There are both physiological and emotional reasons for this. Your adrenal glands produce a hormone called androgen. This hormone stimulates your libido, increasing your sex drive. After menopause, your adrenal glands continue to produce the same amount of androgen as before. In addition to having the same amount of this hormone now, menopause has freed you from the estrogen swings that occurred every month during your menstrual cycle. You have probably been aware of increasing and decreasing sex drive during your menstrual cycle. Now that you are free of these swings, you will probably feel the same sense of desire throughout the month.

Emotionally, you now feel freer to express your sexual self than you did when you were younger and less sure of yourself. You have had more practice now and know what you want. Your inhibitions are probably greatly reduced. In addition, you no longer have to worry about contraception and this can add increased spontaneity to your sex life.

These pluses after menopause more than compensate for the physical changes that take place during menopause. It is, however, a good idea to know what is happening physically that might affect your sex life. Then you won't have to fear these changes so much and you can get the right kind of help should you need it.

After menopause, the cervix, or mouth of the uterus, no longer produces mucus. Your vagina does continue to produce adequate mucus for lubrication during sex, but it may take you longer to achieve that lubrication— the better to enjoy foreplay! The tissues of your vagina thin and shrink somewhat as a result of the aging process and you may need to compensate for this. The best compensation is an enjoyable sex life. Continuing an active sex life will keep your vagina from shrinking excessively. If you do have difficulty during sex—if you experience pain, a burning sensation, or even bleeding—some Vaseline or K-Y jelly will give you the lubrication you need. Don't be afraid to use it. Using it can even be incorporated into the sex act the same way some couples incorporate putting a diaphragm in place.

To help keep your vagina from shrinking too much, you might also try this *stretching exercise*. Insert the first two fingers of one hand into your vagina. Gently separate them to stretch out the walls of the vagina while you rotate them so you touch all walls. If you experience any pain, stop and try again later. Using a little lubricating jelly can usually keep this from being painful.

If you have not had frequent intercourse during menopause, or if you have had no intercourse at all, you will probably find it painful if you suddenly resume your sex life. Your vagina may not stretch enough to accept your partner's penis without pain and even bleeding. The stretching exercise just described will be helpful, but you will probably need to see your doctor. He can prescribe an estrogen cream for you to use temporarily until your vagina has stretched enough for you to resume a normal sex life. It is important that you not be embarrassed about seeing your doctor. This is just one more good reason to find a sympathetic gynecologist.

Karen's husband lost his job while she had menopause. It was a difficult time for both of them. She felt tense and irritable, while her husband felt insecure about his ability to find a new job. They fought continuously and stopped having sex. Karen was miserable because she felt that their lack of sex meant she was undesirable. The couple's problems lasted for about a year, until Karen began to feel better because most of her menopausal symptoms were disappearing. Her husband also found a good job. Their life seemed perfect—except for one thing. They still had not resumed their sex life. They made a few unsuccessful attempts, but Karen experienced pain and did not lubricate sufficiently to have good sex. Her gynecologist was a warm, sympathetic man and she had no qualms about seeing him for something so personal. He prescribed an estrogen cream for Karen to use for a few months. He also showed her how to stretch her vagina gently with her fingers. Very soon, Karen and her husband resumed a satisfying sexual relationship again.

Most women sail through menopause with few problems except for occasional hot flashes. Cynthia says, "Menopause—I hardly knew I'd had one. I felt fine, I kept my life going exactly as I'd always done. The only way I really knew something was going on was that my periods were irregular." Jennifer's experience was typical, too. "I just sort of stopped having periods abruptly and didn't think much about it except that I must be going through menopause. In looking back, I do recall that I'd get very hot sometimes, but it couldn't have bothered me much because I didn't even associate it with hot flashes. A friend who was having hot flashes asked me if I ever had them and only then did I recall getting hot once in a while." Helen said, "I didn't find a thing remarkable about it. I was working very hard at the time and I had no time to think about anything but my job. I guess that's good because it certainly made the whole process uneventful."

Start right now to rid yourself of any ideas you have about menopause as the beginning of the end. Concentrate on how good your life will continue to be. When you feel particularly tense, whether you blame it on menopause or just the ups and downs of everyday life, try this *quick-relaxation exercise.* This little exercise really works and is not as complicated as those where you have to lie down to relax different parts of your body. Who has time to lie down in the midst of a tension-provoking day! You must be seated when you do the exercise because it is necessary to close your eyes and it is not a good idea to try that while standing or moving around.

Close your eyes and gently cup both your hands over them. This is easiest if you lean your elbows on your desk or a table. Your hands will block out light and give you a comfortable sense of being touched. Now concentrate on breathing deeply several times. Take in as much air as you are able to and gently let it out. Repeat this five or six times while you try to concentrate on nothing but breathing. Let your body sink down into your chair and try to feel a sense of calm wash over you. Slowly open your eyes and readjust to the world. You will notice you feel a real sense of having been removed from, and of then coming back into, the world. Do this exercise a half dozen or so times during the course of a tough day. It will truly help refresh you. If you cannot stop to do the exercise, take several very deep breaths when you feel anxious. It is amazing how calming deep breathing can be.

Midlife, even with menopause, can be the most rewarding period of your life. The Caldwell Davis Partners study referred to in the introduction to this book showed that women felt an average of seven years younger than their ages during their entire lives, and that forty to fifty was the peak time for feelings of well-being. During this time, almost 90 percent of the women surveyed felt *fourteen years* younger than they actually were. A surprising 80 percent felt *sixteen years* younger from fifty to sixty. Past sixty, 60 percent felt *seventeen years* younger! That sounds like the kind of positive attitude you will want to take into the years ahead.

ACTION CHECKLIST FOR MENOPAUSE

- Find a good gynecologist.

- See your gynecologist frequently.

- Consider estrogen therapy for severe hot flashes.

- Try vitamin E for mild hot flashes.

- Dress in layers to be comfortable.

- Be responsible about contraception.

- Use home-pregnancy-test kits when you are anxious about pregnancy.

- Do vaginal stretching exercises to assure a good sex life.

- Do quick relaxation exercises when you are tense.

ESTROGEN-REPLACEMENT THERAPY—SHOULD YOU OR SHOULDN'T YOU?

WHAT THE EXPERTS SAY

It used to be common—in fact, almost standard procedure—for a gynecologist to prescribe estrogen for a woman once she started to experience menopausal symptoms. In addition to controlling annoying hot flashes, estrogen was also thought to increase a woman's sense of well-being and help keep her looking young. Suddenly, this bubble burst with the news that estrogen might be responsible for an increasing number of cases of endometrial cancer (cancer of the lining of the uterus). For some time, these nasty suspicions seemed to be confirmed, and estrogen became almost a dirty word. Many doctors would not and still won't touch it, and women were and still are fearful of the consequences of taking it. Now the pendulum has begun to swing back, however, and we are taking a more rational and realistic look at estrogen-replacement therapy. The present attitude is largely the result of new studies done by many doctors. These studies show some interesting and reassuring things about taking oral estrogen. But there is still much to be learned about estrogen and its effect on a woman after menopause. The decision to take it should never be made lightly. The best way to approach such a decision is to consider the risks in *your* particular case and weigh them against the benefits. A desire to look younger should *not* be one of the benefits you consider. There are other, more risk-free ways to improve your appearance.

Dr. Lila Nachtigall, associate professor of obstetrics and gynecology at New York University School of Medicine and director of gynecologic endocrinology at Bellevue and Goldwater Memorial hospitals, conducted a pioneering ten-year study of the effects of estrogen. Though other studies have been done since Dr. Nachtigall published the results of her work in 1977, these new studies have confirmed what Dr. Nachtigall concluded. Here are her answers to some of the most common questions about estrogen-replacement therapy.

What is the most serious long-term risk of estrogen therapy?

Endometrial cancer has been considered the main risk. When estrogen was first given to relieve menopausal symptoms such as hot flashes, it was given alone. The unopposed estrogen did cause the uterine lining, in some cases, to thicken and overgrow. This "hyperplasia," as the overgrowth is called, can be a precancerous condition, though it certainly does not always turn into cancer. Now many doctors give estrogen in combination with progesterone, a second female hormone. The usual sequence is several weeks of estrogen followed by a few days of progesterone. I believe that when estrogen is administered cyclically with progesterone, a woman's risk of endometrial cancer is no greater than normal.

The story is not quite so cut and dried, however. If a woman has an undetected cancer of the uterus or breast, estrogen can make the cancer grow faster. If you are considering taking estrogen, it is crucial to be as certain as possible that you have no cancer when you begin therapy and that you be monitored carefully while you're taking estrogen. It is also possible for a cancer to develop while you're taking estrogen—not as a result of estrogen therapy—and for the cancer's growth to accelerate as a result of the therapy.

Who should take estrogen?

Any woman who is having her life disrupted by menopausal symptoms, primarily hot flashes and night sweats, might consider estrogen therapy. Any woman who has a family history of osteoporosis (a disease, common in older women, in which the bones thin and become brittle and very susceptible to breakage) might also consider estrogen. Estrogen therapy is known to help prevent this debilitating problem.

Who should not take estrogen?

Any woman with a family history of breast or endometrial cancer should probably not take estrogen. A woman with a preexisting cancer of the breast or uterus should also not take estrogen.

How long does estrogen therapy usually last?

If you are taking estrogen for menopausal symptoms, the duration of the therapy is short. It could conceivably be anywhere from several months to a few years. A woman taking estrogen for under two years is probably not at any greater risk of getting endometrial cancer than any other woman. If you are taking estrogen to help prevent osteoporosis, you can expect to take it for ten years or more in order for it to do any real good.

When you stop estrogen, do menopausal symptoms return?

You take estrogen to help your body adjust to the hormonal changes that are going on naturally. You may have abrupt ups and downs in estrogen production or your estrogen production may drop off so sharply that your body has difficulty adjusting. By administering oral estrogen, you can control the amount of estrogen circulating in your body and help make the adjustment process less traumatic. You should not stop taking estrogen abruptly. Your doctor will taper it off gradually, giving your body time to adjust to diminishing levels. By the time you actually stop taking estrogen, your body should be accustomed to the lower level. When estrogen is given this way, symptoms do not reappear.

What can you do to minimize your risk while taking estrogen?

Any woman taking estrogen should see her doctor at least twice a year—some doctors may want to see you more often—for a pelvic and breast exam. This is a must. Unscheduled bleeding (when estrogen is taken in combination with progesterone, bleeding that simulates a menstrual period occurs) should immediately be reported to your doctor.

What do vaginal creams containing estrogen do? Are they dangerous?

If the vagina becomes too dry as a result of menopausal changes, you feel very uncomfortable, and sex can become pain-

ful, if not impossible. Infections can also become a problem. An estrogen cream will definitely help the vagina become more moist and flexible, making you more comfortable and improving your sex life, if that's been a problem. If a dry vagina is your only menopausal symptom, you should probably use the cream rather than take estrogen orally. Oral estrogen circulates in your bloodstream, exposing you to greater risks. It is important to remember, however, that you do absorb some estrogen in your bloodstream as a result of using the cream. Therefore, some of the same precautions suggested when taking oral estrogen are in order here, too. Your doctor should ascertain that you have no reproductive cancer and you should be monitored frequently. Any unusual bleeding should be reported to your doctor immediately.

Are face creams containing estrogen dangerous?

When estrogen is used in a vaginal cream, the cream is almost all estrogen. When it is used in a face cream, it is combined with many other ingredients, so you are getting less estrogen. You will also absorb less through the skin on your face than you will absorb through vaginal tissue. You do, however, probably absorb some estrogen. Since most estrogen-containing face creams are probably prescribed by a doctor, it is important to follow your doctor's instructions for use. Don't use more cream than directed and don't use the cream more often than directed.

C H A P T E R 2

Y O U R   S K I N :
M A K E   I T   Y O U R
B E S T   B E A U T Y
A S S E T

Sometime between the ages of thirty-five and forty, the average woman spends substantial time standing in front of her mirror, fascinated by what she sees. She runs her hands over every tiny line and indentation in her face, wondering if it is soon to become a full-blown wrinkle. What, she wonders, does time have in store for her?

Time does change what your mirror reveals, but consider the following two descriptions of what goes on within your skin and decide which you would rather be facing.

SCENARIO 1

You look into the mirror, studying the face you see reflected before you. Oil sits on your nose, your forehead, your chin, making your face look as shiny as a well-greased muffin tin. You wash your face as often as three times a day, and still your pores fill up with dead skin cells, oil, and other refuse. Some of the clogged pores become infected and form bright red bumps that sometimes become capped with yellow fluid. Other pores become filled with excess oil and skin cells that turn a dark-brown color when exposed to air. Still other pores fill with the same material but appear white on the surface because a thin layer of skin covers the pore opening. Makeup seems to run off, leaving no camouflage for your poor naked skin. Medications are of limited help and tend to irritate your skin, making it red, dry, and flaky. What are you to do?

SCENARIO 2

You look into your mirror and see a clear skin, but one with a few tiny lines around your mouth and eyes. The texture of your skin seems drier and the appearance of your face is not quite as firm as it once was. You find makeup sits in tiny cracks and crevices, but then you discover that moisturizers and sloughers plus a gentler cleanser make your skin look smoother and help makeup slip on more easily. You wash your face only once a day, usually at night, and give it just a hot and cold rinse in the morning.

To those of you who chose scenario 2, congratulations. You have wisely decided not to opt for adolescence a second time! Scenario 1 is a description of typical adolescent skin and the miseries that accompany it. Scenario 2 is a description of mature skin. Actually, both scenarios could be called descriptions of aging skins. A change of life causes the hormone shifts that account for both sets of skin changes. The important thing to remember is that scenario 2 is what you have to look forward to and it is characterized by *gradual,* not drastic, change. So if in adolescence you coped with pimples, excess oil, blackheads, and whiteheads, what are you worried about now? You have already lived through a far worse time. When you compare the two periods, you can't help but decide you are better off now. Remember, too, that when you were in your teens and early twenties, you had very little wisdom about life. Your coping abilities were limited. Now you have had a lot of life experiences and you are far better able to cope with whatever nature has to offer you.

I am not trying to trick you into believing that nothing much is going to happen to your skin as you pass forty and move into your fifties. But I *am* trying to convince you that it is not as bad as you feared, and you will be able to deal with what happens.

What does happen to your skin at midlife? Believe it or not, your skin is one of the most complex organs you have. It breathes, perspires, stretches, and fits you like a glove—at least it used to. It can still do you proud at forty, fifty, and beyond, if you know how to take care of it.

Skin is composed of two distinct layers, the outer

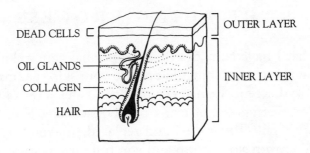

DEAD CELLS

OIL GLANDS

COLLAGEN

HAIR

OUTER LAYER

INNER LAYER

layer, or epidermis, and the inner layer, or dermis. The outer layer provides protection for the inner one, which contains the supporting fibers that give your skin its characteristic appearance. The outer layer consists of many thin sheets of densely packed cells. This layer is constantly growing. The cells that form this outer covering are created at the base of the epidermis where they are constantly being pushed upward to form the outer sheets. Once they reach the outer surface of your skin, the cells are dead and are *shed*, an occurrence of great importance, as you will see later on in this chapter. If you remove, cut, or nick this outer layer, it will grow back. Hair roots and oil and sweat glands are all found here. Damage to this outer layer is relatively easy to repair. It can be fixed "cosmetically." The inner layer is a different matter entirely. The condition of the inner layer gives your skin its basic appearance. As long as this inner layer is intact, the outer layer will look fine, but damage the inner layer, and eventually you have wrinkles and sags that require major repair work to fix. The inner layer of your skin contains elastic fibers and collagen that form your skin's basic support system. Nerves and blood vessels are also present in the inner layer.

THE AGING PROCESS

What I have been describing is normal young skin. As you age, certain things happen to your skin that make it look different. Remember that the outer layer of your skin is composed of many tightly packed cells that are continually being shed and replaced. As you age, new cell growth slows down and you begin to produce a different kind of cell. The cells of aging skin stick together more tenaciously and are not shed as easily as dead cells in younger skin. When layers of dead cells build up, the skin takes on a coarse, dry, and crepey appearance. The cells in older skin also have less ability to retain moisture and this, too, makes the skin appear dry and crepey. Pigmentation in skin increases, and you may notice small dark spots or your skin may become slightly darker all over. In addition to all these changes, your oil glands produce less and less oil.

Drastic as all this may sound, there is much you can do to offset these changes and keep your skin looking smooth and attractive. The outer layer can be sloughed to help remove dead cells. It can be moisturized to replace the moisture you have lost. Your skin can still be "cosmetically" fixed. The changes within the inner layer, however, can be more striking and they are not so easily fixed. The supporting elastic tissues can break down and cause the skin to sag and wrinkle. The aging process causes some breakdown in collagen and elastic tissues, but if this were the only reason for change, you would still look pretty good at sixty or even seventy. Unfortunately, the greatest cause of tissue damage in this layer is overexposure to the sun. I will talk more about this later,

but for now, remember that without excessive exposure
to the sun, you would probably not have much to com-
plain about in the way of sags and wrinkles.

WHAT CAN YOU DO TO COPE?

You have probably been cleansing your skin in a particular way for years. You use a favorite complexion soap
or a cleansing lotion, or, if your skin is very dry, maybe
even a cleansing cream. Now is the time to *reevaluate your
cleansing needs.* Let's start with very dry skin. If your skin
has been dry enough to cause you to use a cleansing
cream (there are very few young women with skin this
dry), you should certainly not change now. If your skin
is normal, you have several options now. If you have
been using a soap, rethink the kind of soap. Is it as mild
as it could be? At this point in your life, you should use
the mildest complexion soap you can find. Several cosmetic companies make good mild soaps you might consider. You might also visit your local drugstore and see
what it has to offer. Any transparent soap is a good
choice or anything that calls itself a mild *complexion* soap.
You can also use any of the numerous cleansing lotions
available at drug and cosmetic counters. Never use the
same soap on your body and on your face. A soap that
cleanses thoroughly for body use would be too strong
for your face, and, conversely, a soap mild enough for
your face won't have the cleansing powers you want in
a body soap. If your skin is oily, it will now become less
oily and you should think of using something milder to

cleanse. A good complexion soap should be fine, perhaps combined with a mild abrasive cleanser used once or twice a week, if you still tend to be quite oily.

In addition to rethinking the product you cleanse with, you might want to *rethink how often you cleanse.* If your skin is dry to normal and you use any kind of soap, you should probably think about cleansing with soap only once a day, preferably in the evening so your skin is thoroughly cleansed of makeup and skin oils. Your morning cleanser can be a mild lotion or even a mild skin toner followed by a splash of hot, then cold, water. Oily skins, unless they are still super-oily, should also be cleansed only once a day with soap, preferably at night. Your morning cleansing should be done with a mild cleansing lotion or light astringent followed with a splash of hot, then cold, water.

This is also the time for you to add a new and vitally important step to your skin routine. *Sloughing* is something you may have read about. You may have seen sloughing products advertised, but perhaps you don't understand the need for sloughing now. Remember that, as a result of the aging process, there is a thick layer of dead cells that clings tenaciously to your skin. Instead of falling off easily, as they used to, the cells stick together and hang on for dear life. To encourage them to disappear, you need to slough your skin. When you were sweet sixteen, a washcloth was an adequate slougher. Now you need something more abrasive. Depending on your skin, you may need anything from a sloughing puff or sponge to a gentle sloughing cleanser used a couple of times a week. If your skin is normal to oily, I would recommend that you try using a facial buffing sponge. You can buy one in any drugstore. Use it daily to encourage dead cells to slough. The best way to use one of these puffs is to incorporate it into your cleansing routine. Rub your soap over the wet puff or drop a little cleansing lotion on it. Massage the puff over your face *gently* in a circular fashion, being sure to cover your entire face. Avoid the area immediately surrounding your eyes.

You can try another method of attack on these dead cells. There are many products on the market called texturizers, refining lotions, or skin tonics, which are all intended to help remove the outer layer of dead cells. Most do so by dissolving some of the cells, leaving your skin looking smoother. It doesn't really make much difference how you slough off these cells, so long as you give nature a little nudge. The best thing to do is to experiment with several different sloughing products and see which work best for your skin. Some may be too abrasive and others may not be abrasive enough. If you are in doubt about what product to use, talk to the saleswomen at several different cosmetic counters. Ask them for recommendations and to explain these recommendations, so you can decide what seems to make the most sense for you. You will probably have to spend a little money to try some of them. It does not make sense to try everything you see, but do try a couple of methods.

I would recommend that you try one sloughing lotion, one sloughing cleanser, and a puff. Try each method for two weeks and see how your skin looks. Settle for the method that seems to keep your skin looking smoothest without causing any irritation or excessive dryness. In general, the fairer your skin, the more sensitive it is and the more careful you will have to be about sloughing. If you have fair, sensitive skin, you will probably find a lotion is best, perhaps combined with a sloughing cleanser used once a week. Normal skins can take a puff daily, and oily skins will need a sloughing cleanser several times a week plus a sloughing puff used daily. If your skin is oily, you could also experiment with a regular-strength sloughing lotion rather than a mild one.

A slougher can make a dramatic improvement in the appearance of your skin. Elizabeth discovered this when she first started using a slougher, on the advice of a friend. "My skin looked coarse and dry with tiny crepey lines here and there," she reported. "A friend suggested I try her sloughing lotion and I did. In a week, I really noticed an improvement. My skin looked softer and had much more of a glow. In two weeks, it began to look red and irritated, especially around my mouth. I checked with the saleswoman in the department store that carried the lotion and she recommended a milder product. I tried this and it's worked beautifully."

Helen's experience was different. "My skin has always been oily and it still is, even in my mid-forties. Lately, I notice my skin seems to have no life. It looks very dull and the oil just sits on the surface, yet my skin seems dry and dull in spite of the oil. I went to one of those stores that sell nothing but beauty products and talked to one of the saleswomen. She recommended a sloughing cleanser and an abrasive sponge. I use the sponge when I wash my face at night. I rub the moist sponge over my soap and scrub gently, then rinse well. Three times a week, I cleanse with an abrasive cleanser. The one I like is an apricot scrub, and I use it in place of my regular soap. I must say, I'm impressed with the change it's made. The texture of my skin is improved, and the oil doesn't sit on the surface; it seems to penetrate my skin and keep it looking moist and soft."

Your skin will respond to sloughing just as well as these women's skins did. But sloughing is only half the story. The other half is *moisturizing*. You have probably been told to use a moisturizer ever since you were sixteen. Most likely, you have been slathering one on for the past twenty years. Moisturizers are the most misunderstood and misused beauty product there is. They have great positive potential, if only you understand how to use them. If your skin is oily, or even normal, you should use a moisturizer judiciously until you are forty or even older. A moisturizer can clog pores, causing breakouts and whiteheads. Most women get into trouble using them on the chin, nose, and forehead where the skin is generously supplied with oil glands. Using a moisturizer here will only cause problems. The neck and the area around the eyes and perhaps just around the rim of the lips are the only places a young woman with normal to oily skin should use a moisturizer. After forty, oil glands slow down and produce less oil. Now you should begin using a moisturizer over your entire face and neck, concentrating on the driest areas. There are dozens and dozens of moisturizers on the market, most of them quite good. Your job is to find the consistency that is best for your skin. If your skin is very dry, a cream will undoubtedly work best. Less dry skins can use a lotion. You may find a cream at night and a lotion for day is a good solution. For day use, you should look for a lotion that is quickly absorbed into your skin, so that makeup can be applied over it easily. If you want your moisturizer to work at optimum efficiency, apply it over damp skin. A moisturizer seals in your skin's nat-

QUICK CARE ROUTINES

DRY SKIN

CLEANSE:
Twice daily, with mild lotion or cream

SLOUGH:
Mild sloughing lotion daily

MOISTURIZE:
Twice daily; cream at night, lotion in the morning

NORMAL SKIN	OILY SKIN
CLEANSE: Twice daily, with mild complexion soap or lotion	CLEANSE: Twice daily, with a good complexion soap; if skin is very oily, use mild abrasive cleanser 2–3 times weekly
SLOUGH: Buffing puff or mild sloughing lotion daily	SLOUGH: Buffing puff or lotion daily. Abrasive sloughing product, 2–3 times weekly
MOISTURIZE: Twice daily with lotion on dry areas only	MOISTURIZE: Daily, at night on driest areas only. If skin is very oily, moisturize around eyes only

ural moisture, keeping it from evaporating quickly. It also penetrates the outer layer of your skin and carries some moisture with it so that your skin looks plumper, firmer, and healthier.

DO THOSE LITTLE MIRACLE CREAMS WORK?

Unless you have been stuck at home for the past five years, you cannot have helped noticing what has been happening at your favorite cosmetic counter. There are dozens of new treatment products on the market now, most geared to the mature skin. They claim to do everything from removing wrinkles to increasing your skin's oxygen supply. Those of us who remember the royal-jelly and placenta and turtle-oil crazes of the past may rightfully wonder if what is going on now is any different. Believe me, there are no miracle creams. Not yet, anyway. We do, however, know a lot more about skin and how it functions than we used to, and because of the increasing interest in health and fitness, cosmetic companies have spent huge sums of money researching new products. As a result, we are now seeing some amazingly effective preparations. Many of the new creams and lotions contain *collagen*. Some contain both collagen and *elastin*.

You can buy a product containing both collagen and elastin for under five dollars or you can pay as much as one hundred dollars for a cream that contains collagen, elastin, and other ingredients. Should you buy the five-dollar cream or the hundred-dollar one? That depends, to some extent, on how much money you have available to spend on your looks. Clearly you are getting something different in the product that costs one hundred dollars—sometimes the packaging alone represents a sizable portion of the product's cost. The real question is, how much more is the expensive product worth?

To answer this question, let us consider what collagen and elastin are supposed to do. Collagen is a naturally occurring substance found in the dermis layer of your skin. It is part of your skin's support system and a part that age breaks down. If there were some way to put new collagen into your skin, you might be able to recapture the firm appearance you had in youth. There is much skepticism about whether the collagen found in cosmetic treatment products actually penetrates the skin's surface deeply enough to cause any internal changes. Some researchers believe it does, but they seem to be in the minority. Most researchers do feel that collagen is an excellent moisturizing aid. The collagen helps seal the skin's surface and prevents excessive loss of natural moisture. It also penetrates the skin's surface enough to carry in some moisture of its own, causing the skin to appear smoother and more moist. Collagen does give the skin a very nice *surface* texture.

Still, you might ask, should I buy the cheaper product or the more expensive one? Unless you have a great deal of money, there does not seem to be any good reason to pay a sky-high price for any product containing collagen, but, on the other hand, you should not buy the cheapest one. Collagen is a tricky substance to work with. You might compare it to the white of an egg. The egg white is liquid, but subject it to heat and the white becomes a solid. Collagen cannot be subjected to heat either. When it is heated it becomes a gel that does not

mix well with anything else. Most companies get around
this problem by carefully formulating their products so
that the collagen is added last and will not be subjected
to any process that will destroy its solubility. Buying a
cream or lotion made by a company with a good reputation is your assurance that the collagen is still soluble
and active in the product. This means you may not want
to buy the cheapest product you can find, but you need
not buy the most expensive one, either.

Elastin is found in many creams and lotions, especially those that claim to remove fine lines. Elastin does
indeed stretch and fill in tiny creases *temporarily*. It will
not smooth out deep lines and it will not do anything
permanently, but there is evidence that it helps give skin
a smoother appearance. Here, too, you need not buy the
most expensive product, just one from a cosmetic company you trust.

You have probably read about creams or lotions that
increase cell turnover in your skin. Why, you may wonder,
should you want to turn over more cells faster? Think
back to the beginning of this chapter. There you learned
that as your skin matures, it produces new cells at a
slower rate and that these cells cling to your skin's surface more tenaciously than they did when you were
younger. These dead cells form a thin, dry, outer layer
that can make your skin look coarse and crepey. Creams
that speed up cell turnover encourage your skin to produce new cells faster and help your skin shed those dry,
dead cells that cling to your skin's surface. This whole
process is very desirable because it leaves your skin with
a much-improved texture. The skin looks finer, more
moist. Moisturizers can penetrate more easily. A product
that promises to increase cell turnover while it moistur-

izes is something you might very well want to try now. You won't have trouble finding such a product in drug or department stores. Ingredients like urea and allantoin are commonly found in these products, though there are other effective ingredients that do the same thing.

We all want to look better. If a ten-dollar jar of cream or a bottle of lotion for twenty dollars really helped, we would all line up. In many ways, new skin-care research has paid off and products are more effective than ever. However, if a product makes wild promises—to remove wrinkles and make you look ten years younger—it is a promise that can never be kept. The only way to get rid of wrinkles permanently is with cosmetic surgery and some of the new collagen injections (more about this in the chapter on cosmetic surgery) and even this combination cannot remove all wrinkles. Creams can help and sometimes make a dramatic improvement, but you must have realistic expectations.

A WORD ABOUT WRINKLE REMOVERS

From time to time, one product or another appears on the market that calls itself a wrinkle remover. These products are all pretty similar. Most are lotions that you apply over the wrinkled area and let dry. You are instructed not to talk or laugh for a minute or two until the lotion dries. The lotion, which is similar to egg white in consistency, dries, leaving a tight film over the wrinkle, smoothing it out momentarily. As soon as you frown, laugh, or squint again, the wrinkle re-forms and cracks the surface of the wrinkle lotion. What you now have is wrinkled wrinkle lotion! Though these products are not usually wildly expensive, they are worthless. They work until you walk out your front door—if that long. The first time your face takes on any expression after applying the lotion, the wrinkle remover is no longer effective.

MIDLIFE ''ADOLESCENCE'' AND HOW TO COPE

Although it is true that as you age, your skin generally becomes drier, you may not experience this drying as a continuum. In midlife, you experience hormone swings that are not as dramatic as those you may have experienced during adolescence, but are, nevertheless, the cause of annoying changes in your hair and skin. Marjorie, a forty-eight-year-old woman, recalls, "When I was forty-five, my skin, which had been clear for years, suddenly began to break out, mostly around my chin. My hair got very oily and I had to begin washing it every day. This lasted for about a year. I was quite upset at first. I thought, 'Do I have to have wrinkles *and* pimples?' I learned to change my routine a little and that helped a lot. I resigned myself to washing my hair daily and I bought an over-the-counter product to dry up the breakouts when they occurred. Actually, it didn't bother me too much because I realized it wouldn't last forever. When I was a teen-ager and my skin broke out, I felt as though it would never clear up."

Cynthia had a different experience. "My skin would alternate between being quite oily and being dry and actually developing little crepey lines under my eyes and on my cheeks. I didn't know how to treat it. By the time I found a routine that worked for the oily phase, my skin would switch and get dry. Things finally evened out and now I have what seems like a pretty normal skin that I can keep looking attractive as long as I use a moisturizer twice a day. My great joy is that after so many years of washing my hair every couple of days, it now looks fine for almost a week. It doesn't begin to look oily until the fifth day after I shampoo it. That's heaven!"

Most women do experience some difficulty with skin and hair during midlife, but the changes are much less dramatic than those that occurred so abruptly during your teen-age years. Gradually, your hormones begin to level out and so does the condition of your skin. You will gradually notice it becoming drier, but you will have plenty of time to experiment with various treatment products to find those that work for you. Most women also find that their hair is not so oily now and they are able to go longer between shampoos. Who isn't glad not to have to spend so many hours a week washing and styling hair!

SHOULD YOU GO TO A FACIAL SALON?

Facial salons have sprung up all across the country offering both facials and customized treatment products. Once again, how much you take advantage of the services these salons offer depends on how much money you have to spend on your looks. Most salons give you a good facial, but you can do the same thing for yourself at home. There are dozens of deep cleansers and masks on the market and these form the basis for most salon facials.

There are, however, some good reasons to visit a good facial salon during this period of your life. If you have had relatively oily skin and still have many blackheads and whiteheads, now is the time to have them removed. Chances are, you can get rid of them for good because your skin will not continue to produce excess oil and form new ones. If you have the time and money, a salon can do a good job of sloughing away dead skin cells and can give you a moist, glowing complexion to take home. If you have a special occasion for which you want to look terrific, do have a facial. But have it a day or two *before* your celebration. A facial can make your skin slightly irritated temporarily and you may get a small pimple or two as a result of the deep cleansing.

Many facial salons now carry their own line of treatment products and some even carry makeup. If you want to experiment with the makeup, do so. You might find some interesting colors, but I would advise against buying treatment products. No salon has the amount of money to spend on treatment formulation or research that a large cosmetic company has, so the salon is clearly not going to be able to offer you anything out of the ordinary. What they generally do is buy wholesale from some manufacturer and resell the products in their salon. You have no idea from whom they buy and many salons, unfortunately, buy the cheapest products they can find, then mark up the price considerably. This is no bargain for you and you may also be getting a poor product.

DO NOT FORGET YOUR BODY

So far, we have talked only about your face. The skin on your body undergoes some of the same changes as your face. Body skin becomes drier with age and needs more moisturizing. You also need to rethink how you cleanse this skin. Some of the things I am going to say about body cleansing will probably shock you, but here goes. You should *bathe less as you get older*. As Americans, we all tend to bathe too much. Most dermatologists will tell you that daily showering, especially in winter, is not good for your skin. It dries it out, causing it to flake and itch. You are probably set in your ways and think you just could not get to work or even out of the house every day without a shower or bath. Try it. Your skin will thank you. You might learn to take what my mother used to call a "spit bath." This kind of bathing takes place in the washbasin rather than the tub. Wash only your face and neck, under your arms and your genitals. If you try alternating a washbasin bath with a regular bath and shower, you will find you have a lot less trouble with dry skin as you get older.

After forty, no bath or shower should be complete without a *body moisturizer*, especially in winter, and if you are tan in the summer. Body moisturizers often are available in your favorite scent, and if you do not have unusually dry skin you might try reinforcing your perfume with a scented body lotion. If your skin is quite dry, and for many women this is the case, it is better to buy a lotion that concentrates on moisturizing rather than on fragrance. Your local drugstore is a good source of body lotions. Read the labels and look for something that contains *urea* or *allantoin,* both considered to be superior humectants (a substance that increases the skin's ability to absorb water). Lactic acid, sodium pyrrolidone, car-boxylic acid, glycerin, propylene glycol, and butylene glycol are also effective humectants.

A body lotion is most effective when applied over slightly damp skin. After your bath or shower, towel dry, leaving some moisture on your skin. Now apply a generous coating of body lotion and let it sink in before you dress. Pay special attention to your elbows, knees, and feet. Skin here can become exceedingly dry and flaky, even raw. You might like to try a *pumice stone or loofah sponge* in your bath. Use either on rough spots to remove flaky skin, then moisturize well. Never use either on raw areas.

THE SUN: YOUR WORST ENEMY OR YOUR BEST FRIEND?

A friend of mine recently came home from a Caribbean vacation. Although she had been gone barely ten days, she returned with a deep tan. When we had lunch the week she returned, she looked at me across the table and said, "Okay, I know you're going to yell at me for getting so tan, but it's too late now to undo the damage I've done all these years and the tan at least looks good while it lasts." The tan did look attractive, but when it began to fade, the dozens of tiny lines on my friend's face seemed even more obvious.

Your skin has a memory, and an unfailing one at that,

when it comes to sun exposure. It remembers every hour on every beach, every walk you have ever taken in the sun. The condition of your skin at forty, and especially at fifty and sixty, reflects perfectly how much time you have spent in the sun. You have probably heard dozens of times that your body skin looks smoother and better than your face as you age. Still, no matter how many times you have heard it, there is no more dramatic proof than looking at any area of your body that has been continuously covered. In these bare bikini days, the only area that still qualifies is your buttocks—and not even this if you have frequented nude beaches. Take a look at your buttocks in a hand mirror. Feel the skin. Don't you wish your face looked and felt this smooth? The *only* reason it does not is because your face has been exposed to too much sun for years. The fairer you are, the more damage the sun has been doing to your skin. Darker skins have more pigment and thus offer more protection against sun damage, but, still, sun damages even the darkest skins over a period of time.

Acceptable sun damage, though no sun damage is really acceptable, is some drying out of the skin and a few tiny lines around eyes and mouth. Unfortunately, most of us don't escape with such minimal damage. What happens to most of us is a more or less total breakdown of the underlying support system of the skin, the collagen and elastin fibers. Once some breakdown occurs in these fibers, skin becomes deeply lined and stretches so that it fits the face not as a glove, as it used to, but as a mitten that seems to belong to a larger sister. Your skin now has loose folds that create sags and bags. If this description doesn't sound very appealing, the reality is even less so! Since fashion is never going to dictate that we walk around with bags over our heads to protect us from sunlight, what are we to do?

Thankfully, in the past five years, more has been done to help you protect your skin than in the past fifty. Research has come up with sun-protection products that really work. Actually, the ingredients and the ideas for these products have been around for years, but it is only lately that the American woman has finally begun to realize the truth about sun and is ready to do something about it. The only thing standing between you and really good sun protection is your own will power. You *must* convince yourself that this summer's tan is neither necessary nor desirable. Don't sit around bemoaning the damage you have already done. Though you may want to resort to some dramatic rescue techniques—cosmetic surgery, a face peel, or collagen injections—you can and should keep the damage from getting worse. Before you enjoy any outdoor activities this summer, *learn about sunscreens,* then use one—all the time. The new sunscreens are extremely effective and since active ingredients must be listed on labels, you will have no trouble finding a good one. Don't use any sun product that lists no active ingredients. A product without active ingredients will give you no protection. Such a product is only a cosmetic. The most effective ingredient is p-aminobenzoic acid or, as it is sometimes called, paba. Next come benzophenone derivatives and p-aminobenzoic derivatives like iso-amyl and glyceryl. Finally, digalloyl trioleate and cinoxate are often found in some products; though they are better than nothing, they are not as good as the first two groups.

Another way to be certain you are getting a good sun product is to *buy one of the new protection-indexed products.*

All such products have a number—from 2 to 15—on the label. Low numbers offer least protection, high numbers offer more, with 15 being a complete sun block. Ideally, we should all wear a number 15 all the time, but many people will not because it does not allow them to tan. A number 7 or 8 will give fairly good protection and will let you get some tan with limited, gradual exposure. If you are unwilling to forgo all tan, you might use a 15 on your face and an 8 on your body. Try to avoid the sun between ten and two, when it is most intense, and, therefore, most damaging to your skin. Remember, also, that the farther south you are when you are exposed to the sun, the more damage the sun will do. There is a good reason why women in sunless northern countries have a reputation for beautiful complexions.

I'm afraid there is more bad news about tanning. Experts used to feel that once you got a tan, preferably by slow, gradual exposure, you built up some natural protection and could take more sun and deepen the tan. New research indicates that a tan is simply visible evidence that you have damaged your skin, even though you may not have gotten a sunburn acquiring the tan. If you really want to protect your skin, you should not tan at all. The pale beauties of the turn of the century were correct in shunning sun exposure.

Even though you may insist on getting some tan in summer, you can do your skin a lot of good by wearing some protection all year long. *Using a makeup or moisturizer* that contains a sunscreen will help enormously. More and more cosmetic companies are adding sunscreens to all kinds of products from lipsticks to shampoos. It is wise to look for these products and use them.

If you are in doubt about whether your favorite makeup or moisturizer contains a sunscreen, read the package label carefully. Most companies want you to know that the sunscreen is there and will tell you somewhere on the product label. If you don't find evidence of a sunscreen, ask the sales representative of the company that makes the product. If your brand does not contain sunscreens, switch; it is worth the trouble.

The changes you experience in your skin after forty, and especially after fifty, will be gradual, especially if you have been sun wise. You need not fear that after menopause you will dry up and wrinkle like a prune. You can adapt to the gradual changes by creating a flexible skin routine. Don't get stuck in a care routine that may have been perfect five years ago, but just doesn't work now. And don't assume it is too late to protect your skin from the sun. It is never too late to start.

ACTION CHECKLIST FOR SKIN

- Reevaluate your cleansing needs.

- Rethink how often you cleanse.

- Begin to use a sloughing product.

- Use one of the Quick Care Routines.

- Bathe less often.

- Try a pumice or loofah in your bath.

- Use a body moisturizer.

- Limit your sun exposure.

- Always wear a sunscreen outdoors.

- Choose cosmetics that contain sunscreens.

HOW DOES SKIN CHANGE AS YOU AGE?

WHAT THE EXPERTS SAY

The Institute for Control of Facial Aging is a unique place. Situated in a dignified brownstone in New York City's Upper East Side, it is probably the only clinic of its kind. Dr. Gerald Imber, a plastic surgeon, and Dr. Stephen Brill Kurtin, a dermatologist, have a combined practice focused entirely on helping women control the aging process. "We don't promise miracles, we offer help," they say, and they do. A visit to the Institute involves a thorough analysis of the patient's skin—with sophisticated new technology that measures moisture content, elasticity, and oil production, among other things—and recommendations for skin care tailor-made to the individual. Both Dr. Imber and Dr. Kurtin have accumulated a vast amount of knowledge about mature skin through their practice that makes them especially qualified to comment on skin problems. Here are Dr. Kurtin's answers to some commonly asked questions.

What factors contribute to skin aging?

Your chronological age, your heredity, your facial habits, and disease all affect the way your skin ages. Anything that affects your body in a negative way affects skin negatively too. One interesting aspect of facial aging is facial habits, the little things we do with our faces that we may not be aware of. Leaning your face on your hand, for example, stretches and pulls the skin. If you continuously do this, you will eventually stretch the skin of your face permanently. Continual frowning is another example. Frowning wears away the collagen and eventually a frown line is produced. Any action, such as smiling or frowning, will wear away the collagen in that area and eventually produce permanent lines. Probably the most important controllable factor in skin aging is sun exposure. Exposure to sun causes the skin to look old before its time. If you examined the skin that had not been exposed to the sun on an eighty-year-old woman under the microscope and compared it with skin from a forty-year-old woman who had a lot of sun exposure, you might not be able to tell much difference! That's how much the sun can affect the condition of your skin. For dramatic proof on your own body, look at the skin on top of your breasts. This skin has probably had a good deal of sun exposure. Now look at the underside of your breasts. Unless you've done a lot of nude sunbathing, you will see a dramatic difference.

Do fluctuations in weight affect the looks of your skin?

Yes, as you get older, your skin loses its capacity to bounce back. If you are going to lose weight, lose it for good. Constant fluctuations can make skin sag. If you plan to have cosmetic surgery and you are overweight, you should lose the weight before having the surgery. If you lose it afterward, you may end up with loose skin again, the very thing you had the lift to correct.

What changes most in a woman's skin as she gets older?

Many things change gradually with the aging process, but after menopause, because of abruptly lowered estrogen levels, skin cells actually change in shape. They become flatter, causing the skin to lack luster. The skin also produces less oil. Moisturizers can help to some extent, but they leave a lot to be desired. Hormones can help considerably. The Institute has developed a moisturizer that contains a small, safe amount of an estrogen hormone, pregnenolone, that improves the luster of the skin and gives it a better appearance. The cream acts directly on the skin and is not absorbed. The cells become less flat and the overall skin appearance is improved. The same effect can be observed as a result of taking oral hormones, though this is usually not recommended.

Do the collagen and elastin creams on the market work?

Not really. Both collagen and elastin are found in your skin, but they are part of the second layer, or dermis, of the skin. For a cream containing these ingredients to do any good, it would have to penetrate deep into the skin through the outer layer, or epidermis. These creams just don't penetrate that deep. It's like rubbing a can with tomatoes and expecting to get tomato juice inside. It won't happen because the tomatoes can't penetrate the can.

What is the best kind of moisturizer to use?

Probably one that doesn't contain mineral oil. Mineral oil is in many moisturizing products and the problem here is that the oil dissolves your natural skin oil so, in essence, you're removing some of the oils you're trying to replace with the moisturizer. It would be better to use a product that didn't contain an ingredient that removes natural oils. Sesame oil is an excellent oil, but it "cracks" easily, meaning it separates easily from other ingredients and so is tricky to manufacture. It is possible, however, to stabilize a product containing the oil so that the ingredients won't separate. When this is done, the sesame oil makes an excellent base for skin creams and lotions.

Is there any such thing as a safe amount of sun?

No. Any unprotected sun exposure is damaging to the skin. This doesn't mean you have to hide in a cave, it simply means you should wear sunscreens with a Sun Protection Factor (SPF) of 15 whenever you are in the sun. After you've played tennis or been swimming or whatever it is you want to do in the sun, sit in the shade to do your socializing.

Are all wrinkles the same?

No, there are three types of wrinkles. The first ones you see are tiny dry-skin wrinkles in areas where your skin is driest—around your eyes, for example. These are "surface" wrinkles, and moisturizers can correct them temporarily. Next you see "movement" wrinkles, those caused by frowning, smiling, or other expressions. These wrinkles originate more deeply in the skin and can't be corrected with moisturizers. Collagen injections are successful in correcting many of these wrinkles. The liquid collagen is injected directly into the wrinkle, causing it to plump out and become considerably less noticeable. Injectable collagen has recently come on the market (under the brand name Zyderm) and it has dramatically changed the success we have treating wrinkles of this kind. There are no problems with collagen shifting position, as there have been with silicone. It's virtually impossible to make a mistake with collagen. There are some problems, however. Approximately one out of every fifty people is allergic to collagen and can't be treated with it. Also, the treatment doesn't last forever. The length of time a correction lasts depends on many things, but some people need additional treatments after eighteen months. You can, of course, have as many treatments over the years as you need. The third kind of wrinkle occurs when skin has stretched and sagged so that it becomes loose and forms a deep wrinkle or fold. Surgery is the only solution for this kind of wrinkle. The skin is cut to remove excess skin and is redraped over muscles and bones so that the folds and wrinkles are smoothed out.

What can a woman do to keep her skin looking good as long as possible?

She can maintain good health habits—eat correctly, follow a regular exercise routine, and maintain the health of the rest of her body. She should be serious about taking care of her skin, and the sooner she starts preventive maintenance, the better her skin will look over her lifetime. It also goes without saying that she should never expose her skin to the sun without the protection of a sunscreen with an SPF of 15.

C H A P T E R 3

H A I R : Y O U R S
C A N A L W A Y S
L O O K G R E A T

Helen stood in front of her mirror, combing out her wet hair. The last rays of a fall sun shone through her bathroom window. The sun shining on her comb caught Helen's eyes. To her horror, Helen saw that the comb was filled with hair. Slowly, she ran it through her hair several more times. When she finished, she took the hair out of her comb and placed it on the sink and began counting the hairs, one by one. When she had reached thirty, she began to cry. Helen had just passed her fortieth birthday and she was convinced that, even though she had never paid any attention to how many hairs were in her comb before, she was losing her hair.

Helen is not so different from many women who mistakenly feel that once they pass forty, they can expect to start losing hair. The fact that you see on the street every day hundreds of middle-aged women with perfectly normal-looking heads of hair does not seem to calm this fear. Women have it all over men when it comes to hair loss, yet we don't seem to enjoy our advantage as much as we should. Irrational fears seem to make too many women worry about losing their hair.

IS YOUR HAIR LOSS NORMAL?

If you are worried about losing your hair, try this little test before you read any further. It will reassure you. Randomly pull out twenty or so hairs. *Normal* daily loss is somewhere between one and two hundred hairs, so you won't miss twenty hairs. Pull them out from different parts of your head—sides, crown, nape, and so on. Now, examine each hair carefully. You may need a magnifying glass for this, but you can probably do the test without one if you have good eyes. At the end of some of the hairs, you will find a little bulblike structure. Other hairs will not have any bulb. If you plucked twenty to twenty-five hairs, two or three or even four should have little bulbs at the end. The rest will not. The hairs with the bulbs are in a final "shedding" phase. These are the hairs you normally lose when you comb or shampoo. On a normal head, you have about one hair with a bulb to every nine without. Chances are, your hair will fall into this perfectly normal pattern.

Although your hair will probably fall within the normal pattern described in the box, you may notice that you lose more hair in the fall. Most people do. Researchers have been unable to explain just why, but most people seem to experience more hair loss during September, October, and perhaps November. That is why Helen may have noticed a few more hairs in her comb than usual, though she, like most of us, did not regularly check her comb. Occasionally, for some reason, we do check, and what we discover can frighten us, usually for no reason.

In order for you to understand what happens to your hair as you age, you need to know how normal hair grows. The growing part of your hair is buried safely under layers of skin. The part that actually produces new hair is called a follicle. The follicle produces the keratin—a kind of protein—that your hair is made of and pushes it out of the follicle until it reaches the surface. The follicle continues to produce new keratin, thus accounting for the growth of the individual hair. A single follicle will continue to produce new hair growth for anywhere from two to six years. People with shorter cycles cannot grow hair as long as those with longer growing cycles. Most of us can grow hair as long as we like. After all, how many people do you know who *want* hair down to their knees?

After a hair has grown as long as it can, it reaches an intermediate stage and winds down from active growth. This intermediate stage lasts just a few weeks. Finally, it reaches a resting phase, which can last up to several months. The hair has ceased growing and will very soon be shed. When it is shed at this stage, it will have the little bulb mentioned before at the root end.

At any one time, roughly 85 percent of your hair will be actively growing and the other 15 percent will be resting or in the intermediate stage. The resting hair is finally shed because a brand-new hair has begun growing and is pushing it out. Hair shedding, then, can be seen as a positive occurrence. Whenever a hair is shed, it is usually because a new hair has pushed an old one out. The normal daily hair loss that you notice in your comb, brush, or on your sink is actually an encouraging sign. It tells you that new hair is replacing old hair and that the growing process is going on.

That is how we all grow hair, but the hair we grow can vary greatly. Some of us have fine, delicate hair, while others have coarse, wiry hair. By now, you probably have a pretty good idea about what kind of hair you have. Fine hair can be difficult to style because it holds curl poorly, but it does have a beautiful silky texture that helps to compensate for its limpness. Coarse hair, unless it is very wiry, is usually relatively easy to style and this type of hair holds a style well. Normal hair, what most of us have, falls somewhere in between and is quite easy to style.

In addition to a texture such as fine, normal, or coarse, every hair has three basic parts. The outer layer, or cuticle, can be compared to the shingles on a roof. The cuticle is composed of dozens of microscopic scales that overlap to form a shiny protective outer covering. Next is the cortex and, finally, the core or medulla. Changes in the cuticle account for most of the problems you encounter with your hair. Excessive use of chemicals in permanent waving or dyeing, excessive heat from curling irons, dryers, or electric rollers all damage the hair's cuticle and make it look dull and unattractive. Damaged

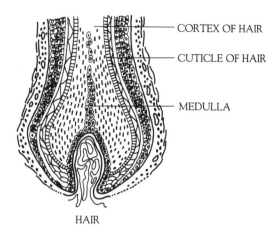

CORTEX OF HAIR

CUTICLE OF HAIR

MEDULLA

HAIR

cuticle results in split ends and flyaway hair. I'll talk more about all this later.

HOW AGING AFFECTS YOUR HAIR

Hair is not unlike skin as it ages. Everything slows down. Hair does not grow as rapidly and is not replaced as rapidly as before so that, at any given time, you have fewer hairs on your head than when you were young, but most of the follicles will continue to produce new hair at a reduced growth rate. The oil glands that supply your hair with oil will also slow down, causing your hair to become drier. Most women are grateful for this, because it relieves them of daily or almost daily shampooing.

There is no denying that a woman does lose some hair as she ages, but her problem, fortunately, is not as acute as a man's, because a woman produces estrogen. Androgens, the male hormones, are present in both men and women. They are responsible for male pattern baldness and for thinning of the hair in women. The female hormone estrogen counteracts the effects of androgens, which is why women do not become bald. As a woman ages, however, she produces less and less estrogen to counteract the effects of the androgens that are always in her bloodstream. With less estrogen to balance the androgens, a woman does lose some hair. Just how much depends on several things.

Your adrenal glands produce some estrogen long after your ovaries have stopped producing it. If they produce enough estrogen, hair loss will be neglible. If they produce very little estrogen, then hair loss may be more significant. There is also another factor involved, however. Some women's hair follicles are much more sensitive to the level of androgens in the bloodstream than others. The level of sensitivity is inherited. For some women, just a slight drop in estrogen causes the hair follicles to shed hair. Other women are not so sensitive, and estrogen can drop off considerably before they notice any change in their hair. If you are concerned about what you have in store for you, consider your mother's hair. Your hormone makeup is probably very much like hers. Keep in mind that your mother's genes are not the only ones influencing your hormone makeup, however, so you will not necessarily duplicate your mother's experience.

Even when hair loss is significant, it is gradual. On a daily basis, you will not be aware of it. It takes years to notice a significant amount of loss. Also, in most cases, hair loss is not substantial until you are well into your sixties. And even then, an attractive style can do a lot to make the hair you have look appealing.

HOW TO COPE

Since hair loss for most women is not significant and is very gradual, loss is not the big problem. Hairstyle is. So many women seem to become trapped at a certain age. By this I mean that they continue to wear a style that looked good on them at one time and never change it. For example, Susan is fifty-one and she still wears her hair in a nearly shoulder-length cascade of curls that looks ridiculous on a fifty-one-year-old woman. Susan remembers how good her long hair looked when she was twenty and thirty and simply will not cut her hair now. Midge, a forty-five-year-old-woman, has chin-length hair styled in a pageboy that she has worn since her twenties. It doesn't look terrible, but it is certainly not the most flattering style she could wear, and it has become boring after so many years.

One of the most important things you can remember about hair as you get older is to be adventurous. *Experiment.* Change your looks. Change your hairdresser. It was important for you to change your looks occasionally when you were younger and it is even more important now. The right hairstyle can keep you from looking dowdy. It can do more to give you an upbeat, young appearance than anything else. Below are five basic styles that look contemporary. You might like to try one of them or you may choose from many others in fashion magazines. I recommend these because they are versatile and easy to care for and have a fresh look.

When you are looking for a new style, don't feel that you can't wear a sophisticated style. Now is the time in your life when you *can* wear something sophisticated. You can wear anything your hair texture is suited to ex-

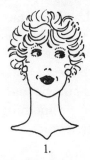

1.

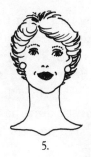

5.

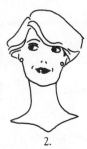

2.

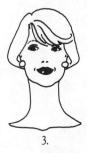

3.

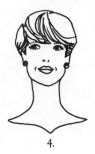

4.

1. For hair that has some curl, or hair that takes a successful permanent, this short, layered style is sophisticated and attractive.

2. For straight hair—especially fine, straight hair—a cut like this is key. It has style, but not too much length. No matter what happens, this look will have a good line.

3. This is a good cut for straight or wavy hair of all textures. The bang softens the line of the cut.

4. A wonderful cut for wavy hair. This style has great sophistication and elegance. A slightly longer version would work for straight hair.

5. This is a wonderful, contemporary cut for almost any texture or any type of hair. Brushed off the face, it makes a lovely frame.

cept very long hair. Hair that is too long drags your face down and emphasizes lines and wrinkles. As a general rule, after forty or forty-five, *your hair should get shorter,* not longer. Be aware of what the new hairstyles are. Read fashion magazines, leaf through the hairstyle magazines that most salons have. Be ready to try something new. If you have had the same style for five years, you should change.

Here are six suggestions that can help your hair help your looks:

- Go shorter, perhaps very short, for easy care and more sophistication.

- Try bangs. They need not be a straight-across chop. Wispy bangs can be soft and pretty, a nice frame for your eyes. You can even try a center part for more sophistication with bangs.

- Try a short style with hair brushed back from your face.

- After forty, don't wear long hair. Chin-length is a good length that provides versatility.

- Consider a permanent to give you more body and volume.

- Consider changing the color of your hair to give your looks a lift (see Chapter 4).

A GOOD CUT, AN ABSOLUTE MUST

Your hair, even if it is terrific, is nothing without a *good cut*. A good cut is not always easy to come by, especially if you don't live in a big city, but it is not impossible, even if you live in the sticks. First, let's talk about the essentials of a good cut. *The right cut is versatile.* It gives you several styling options. It lets you wear your hair fairly curly for dressy occasions and those times when you don't mind fussing with it, and it also lets you wear your hair fairly straight. A good cut allows you to change the part, comb your hair back off your face, or wear it curving around your face. If your hair is chin-length or a bit longer, a good cut should also allow you to have some sort of pinned-up style for evening or times when you want to get your hair out of the way. The essence of a good cut is the line. If your hair is well cut, it will fall into a line as it dries with no urging from you. It should have a "look" even when it is allowed to dry by itself and even if your hair is stick-straight. Remember, the straighter your hair is, the more important a good cut is. Curls hide a multitude of sins.

So, how do you find someone to give you a good cut? This is one time when *making an investment really pays off.* Spend top dollar for a cut, at least the first time. Once you have a good cut, it is not so difficult for another hairstylist to follow the line. If you live outside a large city, it really is worth your while to make a trip into town to get the first good cut. Watch what your hairstylist does, so you can pass along some tips to your local hairstylist. It is a good idea to tell the stylist that someone else will be cutting your hair in the future. He or she can then give you some pointers to pass on.

Don't underestimate word of mouth in finding a good stylist. Ask friends, especially those whose hairstyles you admire, where they had their hair cut. Look in magazines; they credit hairdressers who do models' hair. They also often talk about salons that have branches in major cities. If you are going to a town you don't know, check the telephone book and look at the ads. Who has the most tasteful ad? Call that place. In fact, call a half dozen places and ask how much a cut costs. Ask them if a cut costs the same no matter who does it. You will discover that the best salons charge the most and the best hairstylists at a good salon often get more for a cut than some of the more ordinary stylists. This once, you want the best and you should be prepared to pay for it.

If you have time, it is also a good idea to visit a few salons to see what kind of work is being done, what the clients look like. It may take a little nerve to do this, but remember, it is your hair and you want the best for it, so go ahead and be nervy. You can tell a lot from a quick look inside a salon. If the rock-and-roll music is blaring and you see a lot of stylists in jeans cutting the hair of a very young clientele, this is probably not the place for you. If there are a lot of women with rollers in their hair sitting under dryers, this, too, is probably not the right place. What you are looking for ideally is a mix of clientele, some young, some older, and stylists who seem interested in their work, not in the music and the atmosphere.

Once you have found the right salon and the right stylist, make an appointment for *a consultation*. Most salons will arrange a consultation, often at no charge, if you make an appointment later. Even if there is a charge, it is worth it. The consultation is very important. What you want to accomplish during this visit is an exchange of ideas. You want to see what the stylist thinks would be good for you and you want to give him or her some basic ideas. You should have some ideas of your own. Never just put yourself in the hands of a stylist unless you know that he or she is superb. It doesn't hurt to have with you a couple of pictures that you have torn out of magazines to give the stylist an idea of what you would like to have. Discuss how much time you like to spend on your hair, talk about your hair's texture, whether you want a perm, and whether you color your hair. All these things will affect the cut that is finally chosen.

Your hair texture is crucial in determining what kind of style you should have. Here are some guidelines for various hair types.

FINE, STRAIGHT HAIR

- Never wear your hair longer than chin-length. More length pulls down the style.

- Ask for a blunt cut. It will give hair more fullness at the ends.

- Never layer your hair all over. It will not hold a shape and will be hard to manage.

- Do consider a few layers just around your face to soften the line.

- Consider a body wave for more volume and style flexibility.

- Consider coloring your hair—you needn't change the color dramatically—to give hair more body and a color lift.

FINE, CURLY HAIR

- Wear your hair no longer than chin-length. More length pulls out the curl.

- Don't get an all-over layer cut unless your hair is quite curly. If it is only wavy, your hair probably doesn't have enough body to support a true layered cut.

- Do have a few layers cut around your face. The curl in your hair will help soften features and give you a flattering look.

- If your hair is only slightly curly, a body wave will give it a wavier look.

AVERAGE TEXTURE, STRAIGHT HAIR

- This kind of hair can take most any kind of cut, but don't make it much longer than chin-length. A shorter length is more flattering after age forty or so.

- A blunt cut will give your hair more volume and body.

- If you want a curly style, have a body wave. They are very successful on your kind of hair.

AVERAGE CURLY HAIR

- Do consider a layered cut. It is very flattering for your kind of hair.

- Don't fight the curl in your hair. It is one of your best assets.

- Don't aim for a sleek look; your curly hair isn't meant for this.

COARSE, STRAIGHT HAIR

- Don't have an extremely short cut. Coarse hair is difficult to control when it is too short, especially if it is straight.

- Do consider a body wave to help control your hair. Be certain your stylist doesn't overcurl. You want wave and soft curl, not tight curls.

COARSE, CURLY HAIR

- Don't have your hair cut extremely short. It will be too difficult to work with.

- Don't aim for a super-sleek look. Your hair just won't adjust to this kind of look.

- Don't fight your curl. Trying to make your hair look sleek will never work.

- Cut is very important to your kind of hair. Don't settle for second best. The coarseness of your hair can make a poor cut very unruly.

STYLING OPTIONS

Once you have the right cut, you still have to style your hair. How well you do this can make a big difference in the way your haircut works. Ask the hairdresser who cuts your hair to give you some tips, and watch the way the stylist finishes your hair. Does he or she use a curling iron, electric rollers, or a dryer and brush? What would she suggest you use at home? You will have to do some experimenting to find the best tools for your hair. A *curling iron* is marvelous for fine, straight hair and it is easier to use than a brush and blower. One with "teeth" or "bristles" instead of the conventional clamp will be easiest to use.

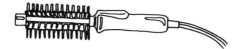

A brush and blower technique is better for hair with some curl and works best for medium-texture or coarse hair. If you have curly hair—either naturally curly or a perm—you might want to let your hair dry naturally for a soft, flattering look. To save time, use a *heat lamp* or a dryer with a *diffuser attachment*. The diffuser—available in many beauty and beauty-supply shops—diffuses the air stream so that your hair can dry without being blown about wildly. There are also some new dryers made especially for this technique. Most have a quartz heating element and a diffuser and are made especially for curly hair.

Learning to use these styling tools takes patience and practice, but do take the time to learn. Nothing looks

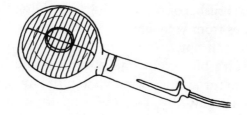

more old-fashioned than hair set on rollers dried under a dryer, yet many women still set their hair this way because they don't know how to do anything else or have not been adventurous enough to try something new.

Set aside a Saturday or a weeknight evening to experiment with your hair. Blow it dry and see how it looks. Rewet your hair and let it dry naturally, then spruce it up with a curling iron for extra polish. Practice with the curling iron. Learn to wind your hair carefully so that the ends are smooth and not crimped. A curling iron with teeth will help grasp hair and keep ends smoother. If you have never learned how to blow-dry your hair, here is a basic how-to technique to follow.

BLOW-DRY TECHNIQUE

Towel dry your hair and part it where you normally would. Clip crown hair up and out of the way, leaving nape hair free. Start drying here at the neckline. Use the dryer and your fingers to dry hair until it is at the "just damp" stage. Depending on how long your hair is, use either a large brush—for chin-length and slightly longer hair—or a skinny brush for shorter hair—and wind small sections of hair around the brush. Wind carefully, so hair is smooth and uncrimped. With hair wound around the brush, continue drying by holding the dryer a few inches from your hair. If your dryer has a "style" setting, use it. If not, turn down the heat volume so that air flow won't blow your hair around so much. Wind hair *under* to turn under, wind *up* to turn hair up. When hair is thoroughly dry, *gently* unwind from brush. Do not disturb the curl until it cools. If you comb or brush the hair while it is still warm, you will pull out the curl. Continue to dry the rest of your hair in the same way. Work up to the crown, then to one side, and the other, and finally the top of your hair, clipping any hair that gets in your way.

HAIR CARE, DO IT RIGHT

Although the way you care for your hair at forty or fifty is not really too different from the way you cared for it at thirty, I think it is important to discuss hair care here because so many women have mistaken ideas about what works and what doesn't. Also, you can't get away with sloppiness now. To look good, you have to take the time and effort to keep your hair in great shape all the time. Your hair needs to be clean and shiny, have a flattering style, and, most of all, be healthy.

WHAT SHAMPOO?

Shampoos *do* matter. There are one or two that might really be better for you than others, so it is worth experimenting. When you were younger, your hair was probably oily and you were most concerned with finding a shampoo that got rid of excess oil. Now your hair is probably not so oily. In fact, you may notice it getting drier. What you want is a shampoo that will leave your hair manageable and shiny. You probably no longer need a shampoo made especially for oily hair. Trial and error is really the only way to find the right shampoo, and, since shampoos are not expensive, you can afford to try several. You will certainly want one that includes some kind of conditioning agent, usually listed on the ingredients list as "protein." The proteins coat the hair, giving it more body and manageability. You will also find that your hair will respond better if you find two or three shampoos you like and *alternate them*. Your hair gets used to the active ingredients in a particular shampoo and may not perform as well if you use it continuously.

CONDITIONING, THE POLISHING STEP

Every woman, yes, *every* woman, should *condition* her hair. How often depends on the kind of hair you have and what you do to it. If you have hair with an average texture and you neither perm nor color it, you can easily get by with *a deep-conditioning treatment once every four to six weeks*. If you have a permanent or you color your hair, you should condition more often. If your hair seems dry and you notice split ends, *a good penetrating conditioner used every two to three weeks is in order*. If your hair seems in good condition, once a month is enough. If you use a curling iron or blow your hair dry several times a week, you definitely need to condition it every three to four weeks. You should also buy one of several products available made to protect your hair against the effects of the heat from dryers and curling irons. Most come in spray form and are easily sprayed on wet hair after shampooing.

If your hair is severely damaged, because you have abused it with too many perms, too much coloring, or too many blow-dryings, you need some serious help. A *hot-oil treatment or a protein pack* will improve the condition of your hair. You should use either every two weeks until your hair is back in good condition again. You should also try to identify what has caused such severe damage to your hair and eliminate whatever it is. Usually severely damaged hair is caused by too frequent coloring or combining coloring with perming when hair is not in good enough condition. Bleaching and straightening are hardest of all on hair, and great care should be taken with any head of hair that has been bleached or chemically straightened. Both procedures, by the way, are best done in a salon by a professional. Most women eventually get into trouble when they do the job themselves.

DEEP VERSUS INSTANT CONDITIONERS

You will see *"deep conditioner"* and *"instant conditioner"* on the labels of many products, and it is important that you know the difference between the two. A deep conditioner is usually left on the hair for fifteen or more minutes, though there are now several products on the market that can be said to deep-condition hair and are only left on for three to five minutes. A deep conditioner is also rinsed out of the hair once it has been left on hair an appropriate amount of time. A deep conditioner actually penetrates the hair shaft; that is, it reaches into the central core of the hair to help replace lost moisture. This results in hair that has more strength, more elasticity, and noticeably more shine and manageability.

An instant conditioner merely coats the hair shaft. It does not penetrate the outer layer. It, too, supplies necessary moisture and gives the hair a better appearance. It helps smooth down the rough spots in the hair's cuticle so that the overall appearance is better. It will make your hair comb more easily and helps control tangles. There is no reason why you should not use an instant conditioner after every shampoo. It takes only a minute, and your hair will stay in better condition. Most instant conditioners are not rinsed out of the hair and remain on until you shampoo again. For this reason, they also help add body to hair. If you have oily hair, be careful about what instant conditioners you choose. You may want to experiment with several to see which is right for you. A water-based instant conditioner is best for oily hair. There are many on the market. Just check the ingredients list to see if "water" or "purified water" is listed near the top. You will also see some sort of protein listed as a major ingredient. When in doubt, experiment.

Do not confuse cream rinses with conditioners. A cream rinse does not condition hair. It coats the hair surface with a waxy substance, making it smooth. It helps prevent tangles and makes wet hair easy to comb. If your hair is fine or oily, a cream rinse is a bad idea. If your hair is coarse, by all means use a cream rinse. It helps soften the coarseness and makes your hair behave better.

Your hair will look good for years. It is the one beauty asset that won't change much over time—except to get gray (solutions for this can be found in the next chapter). The sooner you learn to work with your hair, the sooner you will be on your way to mastering a beauty asset that won't let you down. For most women, if their hair looks good, they feel good. So now is the time to start being your hair's best friend.

ACTION CHECKLIST FOR HAIR

- Experiment with different hairstyles.

- Consider changing your hair to a shorter style.

- Alternate between two or three different shampoos.

- Consider your hair regularly.

- Know the difference between instant and deep conditioners.

- Get the best cut from the best stylist.

- Learn to use styling tools—curling irons, electric rollers, brush, and blow dryer.

GREAT-LOOKING HAIR

WHAT THE EXPERTS SAY

Eva of New York may be the perfect hair salon. It is spacious, soothing, and the client is treated as the valuable person she is. There is no blaring music to jolt you, the stylists are attentive, and being there is an altogether pleasurable experience. You are as likely to see Brooke Shields as an elegant European woman who is staying at the Palace Hotel, where the salon is located, so you can be sure, whether you are sixteen or sixty, that you will get what is appropriate for you. Ralph Damiano is one of the big assets of this salon. He is a whiz with the scissors and I have never known him to give *anyone* a bad cut. He knows unerringly what works for whom. Here is what he has to say about cuts and styling.

How do you make a decision about cutting a new client's hair? What things do you look at?

When a new client comes to me, before I start a cut, I try to spend a few minutes speaking with her about herself and her life-style. I try to determine what kind of woman she is and how she views herself. Is she a working woman, a housewife, both, or neither? How does she wear her clothes, makeup, jewelry? I'll try not only to determine how she should look, but how she views herself. Everyone has her own image of herself, which is not necessarily how others see her. A successful new style has to satisfy not only the client's physical features, but also her personality and the people she comes in contact with. All these ingredients go into making a look work.

What can a new client do to help you find the right style for her?

She needs to tell me what she wants the cut to do—besides make her look beautiful. Does she want it to be an easy, carefree style or does she want something more complicated? It can be helpful to bring a photograph, but she needs to remember that this picutre should represent her physical type and personality. A short, overweight woman of forty should not bring in a picture of Brooke Shields and expect it to be helpful to her.

Are there any particular things you think are not becoming to a woman who is mature?

No woman should ever get trapped into a hairstyle. What looked well in the sixties, when she was twenty, is not going to work for her in the eighties, when she's older. Times have changed and styles have changed. Nothing makes you look more dated than a dated hairstyle. A woman of any age should grow with the times, keeping her hair more tailored as she matures. She should also avoid very trendy hairstyles, which usually only work for very young women. You need to remember that you're no longer cute, you're beautiful now.

What are the best cuts for fine hair?

There are three simple styles that are especially good for fine hair. The "scoop" is a short cut, worn tapered at the neck, then gradually getting fuller at the crown. The hair on top of the head is cut to between three and four inches long. After four inches, fine hair gets too limp. Keeping some fullness on top is the real trick here. It makes fine hair look like more. The sides of this cut are tapered and styled to go away from the face because this is younger looking.

A blunt cut is another safe bet for fine hair. Hair cut one length with a bottom line that is slightly concave, causing the hair to push forward a bit, gives a feeling of volume at the chin and makes a nice frame for the jaw.

Bangs can do wonders for fine hair. They can be cut straight, slanted, or feathered and they add dimension to eyes and cheekbone area.

What kind of cuts are best for very curly hair?

Curly hair is a great foundation for most any hairstyle. Since this hair has volume naturally, it's best to keep the hair closer to the head rather than lift it as you would fine hair. Layers are a must. You should never fight your curl. Show it off, people envy you. A beautiful head of curls will always attract attention. My favorite look for this kind of hair is a full, fluffy waterfall bang, tapered at the cheekbone area, then the rest of the hair is cut to curve around the ear and fall longer in back. From the front it looks like a beautiful short cut followed by a halo of hair.

What should you avoid if your hair is very fine?

You should avoid a long, multilayered style. You should also avoid any style with a complicated routine. You'll always wonder if the end justifies the means! Remember that fine hair is too limp to hold exaggerated lines or flamboyant angled cuts. You should also be careful not to overdo the chemicals you use on your hair. For example, a permanent combined with lots of highlights is bound to end in trouble.

What should you avoid if you have very coarse hair combined with lots of curl?

Most people who have coarse, curly hair seem to want it to look flat and straight—an impossibility. Success with this kind of hair is just a matter of accepting your texture for what it is. You should never opt for a sleek, smooth style. Use your curl and let it give your hair lots of attractive volume.

CHAPTER 4

HAIR COLOR:

A

CONTROLLABLE

ASSET

The day after Helen's fortieth birthday, she had her brown hair tinted strawberry blond. Behind this simple act two powerful emotions were at play. Helen had the classic "fear of forty," and she had also invested her hair color with the power to make her look young and pretty and feel good about herself. Helen is not alone. Most women feel their hair color has a lot to do with how attractive they are perceived as being. Think of all the clichés about hair color—blondes have more fun, gentlemen prefer blondes, redheads are passionate. In truth, hair color does have a lot to do with looks, and today there is almost nothing you could want in the way of a new color that you cannot have. The only problem is deciding what you should or should not try. Since it is easy to learn from the experiences of someone else, consider the stories of these women.

Cynthia had been having her mouse-brown hair highlighted golden blond for ten years. She had always liked the look, but she began to feel that it was not becoming anymore. She had some gray hair and she felt that with her own natural brown, the gray, and the highlighted blond, her hair was beginning to look like the "coat of many colors." She had also been going to the same colorist for ten years and she felt no enthusiasm existed between them anymore. She had been expressing boredom and dissatisfaction for about a year, and the colorist had no fresh suggestions to make. Cynthia finally decided to go to someone new for a consultation and see what other options she might have. The colorist she chose was the head of the color salon in a leading department store. He suggested that Cynthia stop highlighting her hair because it did, indeed, look dated and was unbecoming because her gray hair was so much lighter than the gold highlights. He suggested a one-color *tint* in a golden red-brown. Cynthia had been a redhead as a child and still had the ruddy complexion and freckles of a redhead and the suggestion seemed like a good one to her. She made an appointment the following week, after asking a lot of questions about what she would be getting in for in the way of upkeep with the new color. Cynthia loved her new look. It gave her just the lift she was looking for; and the upkeep was not a surprise, because she had discussed it before making her decision.

Cynthia's story is ideal. She did all the right things and had a predictably happy result. Before you decide that changing your hair color is as easy as ABC, consider what happened to four other women.

Marian's dark-brown hair had been getting grayer and grayer, and although she didn't especially like it, she had not done anything about it. Suddenly—unfortunately, the way we often make important decisions—she decided she could not stand it any longer. She went to her local drugstore and surveyed the aisles of hair-color products. Settling on something called a *semipermanent* color, she picked a dark "ash" brown shade. She didn't know what the ash meant in the shade description, but she liked the picture on the box, so she bought the product. She went home and colored her hair, following the instructions in the package. At first she was pleased with the results, but as the weeks went on, Marian thought her hair had a greenish cast in certain lights. Finally, to her horror, she was sure her hair looked green. She bought a second application of the same product and tried again. At first it looked fine, but, in a few weeks, the same thing happened. This time, Marian bought a darker shade and tried a third time. She hated the results. Her hair looked as though she had colored it with brown shoe polish. Distraught, she finally went to a salon and explained her problem. The colorist told her that she had too much gray in her hair to use a semipermanent, especially an "ash" shade. When the color began to fade, the ash pigment, which has a greenish tint, remained and made her gray hair look green. He suggested that Marian use a permanent tint, because it was the only thing that would completely cover gray. He explained that she could do it herself or have the salon do it. She had had enough of at-home experimenting and she decided to let the colorist do the job. He tinted her hair a soft deep brown that looked natural and covered the gray. Moral: Try to educate yourself a bit before you jump into hair color. If you have problems, go immediately to a good salon. Don't try to solve the problem yourself.

Barbara was tired of her mouse-brown hair and the even mousier gray that was beginning to creep in at her temples and over her brow. She had pretty hazel eyes and fair skin, so she decided that she could be a successful blonde. She went to the closest drugstore and picked a product with a pretty blonde's picture on the box. The picture showed shimmery, pale-blond hair and Barbara became excited at the thought of transforming her own dull color into something so lively. She did exactly as the directions told her—but her hair turned a brassy orange color. Horrified, she immediately went to her neighborhood salon and told her troubles to a friendly colorist. The colorist explained that the color on the box and the colors on most color charts show the color of the product on *white* hair. Most of us don't have white hair, so we don't get the same results as the model on the box. Some products tell you how many shades a color lightens so you can gauge the amount of change, depending on your natural color. It is always best to do a test strand—recommended in most product instructions—before doing your entire head. This way you can stop trouble before you have a headful.

Doris had brunette hair and skin coloring and was bored with it. Like so many of us, she felt the grass was greener on the other side of the fence and she wanted to be a blonde. She, too, went to the drugstore and checked out what was there. By dumb luck, she picked a product that turned her brunette hair a fairly pretty shade of deep golden blond. She was happy with the color, but her complexion looked unattractive next to the blond hair and her dark eyebrows looked like two exclamation marks. Probably worst of all, in a little more than two weeks, she could see dark-brown roots. The third week, Doris was forced to redo her color job. Doris had not foreseen how much upkeep there would be in making such a drastic color change, and she had not given much thought to whether her new color would work with her skin coloring and brows. Both of these features are important considerations when you change your hair color. Given the problems Doris had, she decided that she would switch from such a light color to something that gave her natural color a lift, yet did not require such frequent touch-ups and also was more flattering to her complexion.

Lois had a very common problem. Her hair had been a nice soft blond in her teens and twenties, but since her late thirties, she had noticed that her hair seemed to lose its life. The color was drab and faded. She was afraid to attempt anything too drastic, so she tried a *rinse*. It helped a bit, but it was too much trouble to apply after every shampoo. Next, she tried a semipermanent and loved the results—for the first two weeks. After that, she felt her hair looked exactly as it always did. After doing a little research, she settled on a shampoo-in product that was close to her natural color, but gave just a little lift. Lois learned that you have to be a little adventurous to get the results you want.

These women give you an idea of the most common hair-color problems and how easy it is to fall victim to them. With a little patience and thought, you can avoid all of them and end up with just the color you want.

GRAY: SHOULD YOU LOVE IT OR COLOR IT?

Though gray hair can be enormously flattering, most women hate it and prefer to color it. It would be a lot easier—and cheaper—to accept what nature gives us, but it is difficult to fight a society that equates gray hair with age, and consequently with unattractiveness. Like many of the things society leads us to believe, this is not necessarily true. Many women begin to go gray in their early thirties, sometimes even before. Still, knowing this may not help you love your gray hair. Much of the decision to color or not is purely a matter of taste, but there are certain times when color seems to be the best option.

Unless you fit into one of the categories described in the box on the next page, you don't have much to help you make your decision, except your own personal feelings about your hair color. Like cosmetic surgery, or any other fairly serious beauty step you take, coloring your hair will not change your life. If you invest hair color with powers it does not have, you are in for trouble. If you believe becoming a blonde or a redhead will make

COLOR YOUR GRAY HAIR IF . . .

You begin to get quite gray while you are young. This kind of early graying is usually inherited and can make a young woman feel self-conscious.

It affects your job potential. If it is important for you to project a young image at your job—you work in a young person's field, you are an entertainer, or older people are not perceived as being able to do your job—then it is important to use hair color as an aid to looking young.

The gray hair is unbecoming. Gray hair is often quite becoming, even striking, but sometimes, usually on people who have very dark hair and sallow complexions, gray hair muddies the complexion and is unflattering. A new color can help enormously.

Your gray is more yellow than gray. Yellowish gray is not flattering to most complexions.

your husband appreciate you more or make you happier with your job, watch out. You are not being realistic. On the other hand, a fresher color can give you a new perspective on your looks. It can cheer you up, make your makeup look more flattering, and give you new clothes-color options. If you make the decision realistically, a color lift can give you great pleasure.

There are many ways to dip into hair color. Picking

something that won't create a drastic change is the best way to start. Here are your options from the least drastic to the most.

THE SEMIPERMANENTS

A semipermanent color lasts for a limited number of shampoos—usually six to eight—and fades away gradually. The product will tell you through how many shampoos you can expect the color to last. Most semipermanents are meant to color a limited amount of gray hair or to give a lift to your natural color. They will not drastically affect the color of your hair. If your hair is not terribly gray or you just want a few highlights, a semipermanent is a good choice. Another plus is that you can do the job quite easily at home. The foam-in products are especially easy to use. Most of the major hair-color companies make a semipermanent color and provide excellent instructions.

Semipermanents will not lighten your hair. They can make it a couple of shades darker and they can add red or golden highlights to light- or medium-brown hair. When picking a color, pick a shade close to your natural color with either red or gold highlights. If you are covering gray, it is best to pick the color closest to your own. When in doubt, always pick a slightly lighter shade. It will be more flattering than a darker one.

If your hair is quite gray and you use a semipermanent, don't expect it to cover the gray completely. Be very careful about what shade you pick; any "ash" color can potentially leave a greenish cast in your hair as the color fades. As the original brown color begins to wash out, the ash pigment is all that remains, and on gray hair

PICK A SEMIPERMANENT
COLOR IF:

You want to do the job yourself

You want to cover only a little gray

You don't want a drastic color change

You want to take a first tentative hair-color step

it takes on a greenish look. In general, if your hair is 50 percent gray or more, a semipermanent is not a good choice. You should consider a permanent tint, if you want to cover this much gray successfully.

HIGHLIGHTING

Highlighting is another way to try out a new hair color without making a drastic commitment. When hair is highlighted, tiny strands of hair, mostly around your face, are lightened with bleach. The overall effect makes hair look lighter and livelier. Sometimes the highlighted hair is tinted with a second product to give it a deeper blond or reddish tone. Highlighting with bleach can look very attractive on light- to medium-brown hair. It is not recommended for dark-brown hair. The contrast between the highlighted hair and the dark natural color is too great. Highlighting can be done at home with a kit sold at most drug and cosmetic counters or in a salon. If you plan to do it yourself, start with only a few highlights. You can always add more later if you like the look, but if you make a mistake and start with too many, you will have to wait until they grow out.

The newest and most flattering way to highlight hair is not with a bleach—though many salons still use only a bleach—but with a permanent tint. Using any number of medium-blond to red-blond shades, the colorist can achieve lovely results. Even brunettes can have hair highlighted this way because a deep-blond or very light-brown tint that won't contrast harshly with the deeper natural color can be used. This kind of highlighting can be done only in a salon.

If your hair is light to medium brown and you are just beginning to turn gray, highlighting can be a successful way to conceal the gray. Gray hair blends in with the highlighted hair giving you a flattering allover lighter effect. You may be able to get away with this minimal hair coloring for several years before you have to switch to a permanent color.

Highlighting is permanent. It will not fade with shampoos and must grow out. If the job is skillfully done, it should last two to three months. Sometimes, on light-brown hair, it can last four to six months. You should not have hair highlighted more often than every two months and if you do it this often, you should only have the hair around your face touched up.

CHOOSE HIGHLIGHTING IF:

You want to conceal minimal gray

You have light- to medium-brown hair

You want minimal upkeep

You don't want a drastic change

PERMANENT COLOR

Permanent hair color offers you the biggest range of colors, but is also the most demanding solution. You need to choose carefully and know what you are getting into in the way of upkeep.

Most *good* colorists will not advise you to go more than two shades lighter or darker than your natural hair color, especially if you are coloring your hair for the first time. This subtle change will be more flattering and much easier for you to get used to than a more radical color alteration. Almost all permanent color is mixed with peroxide and thus can lighten or darken your hair any number of shades. But that doesn't mean you should jump in and drastically lighten or darken your hair. Start slowly. You can always go lighter or darker next time.

If you want to hide the fact that you are getting gray, pick the color closest to your natural one. If you would like a color lift, lighten your natural color a shade or two. In general, it is more flattering to lighten as you age. Going darker tends to add a harsh contrast between skin and hair. Darker colors also tend to look more artificial. If you are coloring for the first time and want a lift rather than to hide gray, take your cue from nature. Nature seldom makes a mistake with coloring. If you have brown hair or "dishwater blond," you can get a nice boost from a deep-blond color. Take a look at your natural color in the sunlight and see what kind of highlights you have. If you have golden highlights, pick a color with gold; if you have reddish highlights, pick something with red in it. Stay away from ashy colors.

They tend not to be as flattering as gold or red tones. (Ash shades have no red or gold highlights.)

If you have never colored your hair before, it is always best to have it done in a salon the first few times, because root touch-ups are tricky to do yourself. Some salons will tell you what color and brand they use, so you can do it at home next time. If you stick to a color close to your own, doing it yourself can be successful. If the color is much lighter or darker, it is best to let a salon do the job.

If an at-home color job is what you are after, the most successful way to do it is with a shampoo-in color. This is permanent color, but you use it much like a shampoo. You leave the color on your hair for the allotted time— usually about a half hour—and then just rinse it off. Your hair is then shampooed and colored in one step. If you are not aiming for a drastic change and you follow the directions carefully, this can be a happy choice. It is certainly better than a color that must be touched up on the roots only. Some women are able to do this at home, but most find it very difficult, especially for the hair in back. If you have a dependable, handy friend, you may be able to surmount this problem, but remember, if you need a touch-up and your friend is not available, you have a problem.

Though a shampoo-in color is definitely the best at-home choice, there are some problems you need to be aware of. When used over a long period of time, the shampoo-in color tends to build up in the ends of your hair, because the ends are usually more porous than the rest of your hair and absorb more color. There are two things you can do about this. First, have the ends of your hair trimmed regularly to get rid of the porous, split tips. Second, apply the color to all but the ends of your hair. About ten minutes before you rinse the color, apply it to the ends. This way, the ends are not subjected to as much color as the rest of your hair and you get a more even look. Another way to avoid trouble is to wear your hair quite short. Short hair usually stays in good condition and you need not worry about porous ends.

If you have any problems with home hair color, don't try to solve them yourself—this usually produces disastrous results. Go to a good salon and tell the colorist what product you have been using and what the problem is. This way, you will get a professional solution.

THE GENTLE PERMANENTS

Cosmetic companies are always improving their products, and hair colors are no exception. Recently a new group of permanent hair-coloring products came on the market that contain no peroxide or ammonia. Product labels will always tell you if they don't contain these ingredients. This makes them very gentle and easy on the hair, and the colors are subtle and exceptionally attractive. They will lighten only a shade or two and do not produce drastic changes. The results are permanent; that is, the color will not wash out or fade appreciably. It must grow out. These colors are so new that not all salons have them. You may have to ask around before you find a salon that uses them, but if you want a subtle, gentle lift, they are ideal. They also leave your hair in beautiful condition.

CHOOSE A PERMANENT COLOR IF:

You want to color a lot of gray

You want a definite color change

You are prepared for the upkeep

You are prepared to condition your hair regularly

COLOR IS A COMMITMENT

Though hair color can give you a glorious glow and can be one of your best beauty tools, it *is* a new responsibility. Once you start coloring, you must continue. Roots will need to be touched up every four to five weeks, or slightly longer if the new color is close to your own. All this can be time-consuming and expensive. Helen, who colored her hair strawberry blond, found that out the hard way. She impetuously decided to make the change and was shocked to find that it would cost her almost $500 a year, including the color, tips, and transportation to and from the salon. Fortunately, Helen loved her new color and did not mind, but for every Helen, there are several others who wish they had never started the whole thing. You must be prepared to spend a good hour to an hour and a half every time you have your hair colored; and you should also figure out how much you will spend over the period of a year so you know exactly what to expect.

In addition to the cost in time and money, coloring means more *conditioning*. Even the gentlest colors make your hair more fragile and vulnerable to breakage and split ends. You will need to condition your hair every week or so once you start coloring to keep it in shiny, healthy condition. You will also need to be more careful about what else you do to it. Hair that has been colored must be treated gently. It is not a good idea to have a permanent and to color your hair. It can be done, but it is tricky. If you want to have a permanent, you *must* use a permanent solution made especially for color-treated hair. You should always do a test curl to see if your hair is in good enough condition to take a curl successfully. If you can afford it, go to a salon for your permanent. The results will be more predictable than at home. A permanent must always *precede* hair color because the waving lotion lifts out some of the hair color. You should wait at least a week between a permanent and coloring.

Heated appliances such as curling irons and electric rollers and dryers are hard on colored hair, so use them judiciously. A conditioner helps repair the damage done by heat appliances, but you will need to treat your hair with extra care once it has been colored. If it has been colored *and* permanented, curling irons or electric rollers are not a good idea.

You may find other precautions necessary with colored hair. Sun will lighten your color very quickly, so if you spend a lot of time outdoors, keep your hair covered with a scarf or some sort of hat. If you swim in salt or chlorinated water, rinse your hair immediately afterward.

MAKEUP

It is possible to change your hair color without changing your makeup, but, generally, some change in makeup is flattering. Once you have adjusted to the new color, take a long hard look at your makeup to see if you really think it is as flattering to the new hair color as it was to the old. Experiment a bit with slightly different colors to see if something new might not be more becoming. If you have lightened your hair color, chances are you need to lighten, or at least soften, your makeup colors. Even if you have darkened your hair, a softer makeup palette will probably be more attractive. The most important thing to remember is to pay attention to your makeup. Don't assume that what you wore before will work now. It may not.

WILL THE NEW COLOR MAKE YOU HAPPY?

Any change, even a change you desire, can be frightening at first. You are used to seeing your hair one way, and even though you may not like it that way, it is familiar. Changing it may make you feel strange at first. Don't expect to fall in love with a new color immediately. You might, but if you don't, it doesn't mean you have made a mistake. Give yourself some time to adjust to the change, to see it in all lights, to try it with your familiar but well-loved clothes. If you have thought carefully before you made the color switch, you will probably be happy with it, even though it may take a bit of getting used to. But if you have given the new color a fair chance and still don't like it, by all means don't settle. It is not difficult to change color, especially permanent color. You can try a slightly darker or lighter shade, or one that is more red or blond. You should give each of these successive changes the same getting-used-to period as the first color you tried. Over a period of time, you are bound to find just the color that makes you happy and is flattering.

ACTION CHECKLIST FOR HAIR COLOR

- Start changing your hair color slowly and gradually. Don't make dramatic changes.
- Be objective about gray hair. Maybe coloring isn't your most flattering option.
- When you first color, start with a product that will wash out gradually, rather than grow out. It allows for first-time mistakes.
- Don't lighten or darken more than two shades.
- Have your hair professionally colored, if you can possibly afford it.
- If you have any coloring problems, don't attempt to solve them yourself. Let a professional help.
- Don't opt for the coloring clichés of blond or red unless your skin color works for your choice.

HOW TO APPROACH COLOR

WHAT THE EXPERTS SAY

Bob Prestianni of Pipino Buccheri salon in New York City is unquestionably one of the best colorists in the country. He knows his business and has an uncanny knack for recommending just the right shade for first-time color ventures. The salon itself is attractive and pleasant to be in, and the service is marvelous. Here are Mr. Prestianni's answers to some of the most common hair-color questions.

How do you decide what kind of color will be flattering when you see a woman for the first time?

I look at her skin, face, and makeup. I can tell from her makeup what sort of colors she inherently likes. I also consider the texture of her hair and what kind of color change it can sustain. I feel that nature never makes a mistake when it comes to hair color, and any new shade I recommend will be within the range of the natural color. As you age, however, I do believe it's more flattering if the hair gets slightly lighter. But it's important for a woman to remember that too light can be just as harsh as too dark. You have to pick a balance between the natural color and something that's just a bit lighter or darker.

Do you think a woman should ever make a drastic hair-color change?

NO! I don't believe the hair color should change more than two shades in most cases.

What is the best approach for covering varying amounts of gray?

When a woman comes to me and says she wants to get rid of her gray, I study her hair to see what the darkest color is—her natural color—and what the lightest color is—the gray. Then I try to hit a balance between these extremes. The right new color for this woman is somewhere in between the lightest and darkest colors on her head.

What kind of color covers gray best?

A semipermanent covers fairly well if hair is not too gray and not too coarse. The semipermanent lasts from five to six weeks, but most women find they are not terribly happy with the way their hair looks after the first few weeks. Generally, they switch to a permanent color after they get used to the idea of coloring their hair. Gold and red tones are a better choice for semipermanents. The ash colors tend to have a greenish cast when they wear off. If the hair is quite gray or if the texture is coarse, I recommend a permanent color. It's really the only successful way to cover gray for this kind of hair.

Who is the best candidate to become a redhead?

The woman who was a redhead when she was a child is the best. She has the kind of ruddy complexion that goes well with red hair. Red brings out the color in your skin, so it's important that you have the right color. Most women who have a ruddy complexion can wear some shade of red. Red is the one color that should not be tried at home. It's very tricky to get the right, soft shade. The nice thing about red, though, is that no two are alike. It's a very individual color.

Who is the best candidate to become a blonde?

Any woman who had light-brown or blond hair as a child is a good candidate for becoming a blonde in later life. Anyone with hair darker than medium brown should not attempt to become a blonde.

How can you avoid the "shoe polish" look dark colors sometimes have?

The trick is to not get into very dark colors. This problem usually happens when a brunette with a lot of gray tries to match her natural dark color. It's best to pick a new color that's a bit lighter than the natural color. It will be more flattering. If you're doing the job yourself, especially with a shampoo-in color, watch out for the ends. Don't put color on them until you're almost ready to rinse it out. Just leave it on the ends for only a few minutes and you won't get that unattractive dark buildup.

What do you find to be the most common hair-color problem?

Hair that's in poor condition is the problem I see most of. When you color your hair, you must, first of all, pick the right shampoo. Be sure you use a shampoo that's mild and made especially for color-treated hair. Next, you must condition your hair. You should use a good conditioner once a week to keep colored hair in really first-rate shape. Remember that you can't treat colored hair like regular hair. You'll get into trouble if you do.

The next most common problem is blondes that are too blond. Many women who have been two-process blondes (hair is first bleached to a very pale shade, then, in a second process, a toner is applied to achieve the finished color) for years, come in and want a change, but they don't really want to give up this very blond look. When I give them a darker, much more flattering shade of blond, or even a light brown, they are very unhappy because they have this blond image in their heads. It's why I stress that picking a color that's too pale can be just as harsh as one that's too dark. That very pale two-process blond look isn't flattering for most women. It's too light and it has no life.

C H A P T E R 5

M A K E U P :

L E S S I S

M O R E

I had lunch recently with a friend I hadn't seen in several months. As I sat across the luncheon table from Ellen, I noticed she was wearing too much makeup. As the sunlight flooded into the restaurant, I could see that her tawny blush had collected in the tiny lines and little dry-skin flakes across her cheeks. The brown eye shadow on her eyes was creased in the folds of her lids. Little trickles of lip gloss seeped into the minute lines on her upper lip.

Ellen is very pretty and has always worn makeup that accented her lovely, big hazel eyes and high cheekbones, but now, at forty-four, her delicate fair skin was showing some subtle signs of aging. Like many of us, Ellen had been applying the same makeup for years, without paying much attention to how it really looked. Sometime around age forty, we need to throw away all our old makeup habits and start afresh, taking into consideration just how we look now. Much of what you have been doing with makeup may be fine; the important thing is to take an objective look now.

I have another friend, Fran, who is also typical of many women around forty. Fran never used to wear much makeup, but when she began to realize she did not look as young as she used to, she tried to compensate by using more makeup to "hide" behind. This never works. Rather than hiding flaws, too much makeup only accentuates them. Don't get trapped into either of these mistakes—too much makeup or the same old thing. After forty, the most important thing you can learn is that *less is more*, truly!

WHAT DO YOU REALLY LOOK LIKE NOW?

Even if you feel happy with your makeup, try this little experiment. It will help you get a fresh perspective on the way you look now. With a clean face and freshly washed and styled hair, sit in front of a mirror with good, but not harsh, light. Apply only mascara and lipstick and, if you have very pale brows, a little brow makeup. This minimal makeup will keep you from looking washed out, but won't really change or emphasize any particular feature. Study your face. Laugh, smile. Take a hand mirror and look at your profile. Back away from the mirror so you can see yourself from the waist up. Talk, laugh, smile, and really look at the "stranger" in the mirror. What do you notice about her most? Does she have a nice smile, a beautifully shaped nose, high cheekbones, a soft, pretty mouth? Don't look for the feature you liked best when you were younger—it may no longer be your best feature. Something else may seem more appealing now. Also, don't focus on the feature you like least. If you focus only on what you don't like, you won't see anything else. Remember what you like best about your face. That is what you will want to emphasize when you plan your new makeup. Another way to obtain a fresh idea of your looks now is to try to catch yourself, *quickly*, in a shop window as you pass by. Pretend that you are glancing at a stranger. What do you see that you like?

Now pull out the family album or whatever old pictures you have of yourself over a span of years, say from the time you were twenty-five up to now. You're going to look at these pictures for changes that have occurred over the years. But before you start studying them, remember what you saw *now* in your face that you liked. It is important that you not lament about what has changed. Remember that, in many ways, you may look a lot better now than you did fifteen years ago. The life experiences and self-confidence you have gathered over the years are reflected in your looks. The way you carry yourself, the expression in your face are probably quite different from what they were fifteen years ago—and probably a lot better. What you want to learn from old pictures is what has changed physically, so you can be realistic about making up your best features now. If you discover, looking at your pictures over a span of years, that your eyes are no longer your best feature because they are not as big as they once were, or that you have gained weight and your cheekbones are not as prominent as they once were, don't accent these features with makeup. Instead, play up a pretty mouth or stop using such deep blush on your cheekbones. *Respond honestly to the changes in your looks.*

THE RIGHT MAKEUP FOR NOW

The makeup you considered essential ten, even five years ago may not be necessary at all now. Here is a checklist that I think is essential for anyone with mature skin. You will notice that some surprising things are missing, and some new things may be added.

WHAT YOU NEED NOW

Several cosmetic sponges

Blusher, either powder or cream

Mascara

Brow makeup (either powder or pencil)

Eye shadow (powder or cream)

Pressed powder

Lip pencil

Lipstick

The biggest surprise on this list is probably the lack of foundation. Believe it or not, foundation may be making you look older than you really are. I can almost guarantee that it is if your skin is dry and delicate. Foundation gets into tiny creases and sticks on dry-skin flakes. If you were not wearing foundation, chances are no one would notice these small flaws. That is why you should try an experiment. I am not suggesting that you leave the house this way; just try it now. *Make up your face without foundation!*

First, apply a good moisturizer and let it sink into your skin. When it is completely absorbed, make up the rest of your face as you normally would, then *finish*—and this is the important step—with a little *pressed powder*. For the best finish, apply the powder with a *slightly damp cosmetic sponge*. There are a few pressed powders on the market that are made to be applied dry or with a damp sponge. One excellent one is made by a French company whose products are popular in the United States.

The damp sponge is the secret. Powder applied this way does not look pasty or flaky. Pick a nice warm shade to add life to your face.

Look at your face objectively, especially about a half hour after you have made up, and decide whether you look better this way or with your usual foundation. The only skin that really looks better with a foundation is oily skin—then you need a water-base, oil-blotting foundation—or skin with acne scarring. A good foundation will help conceal the scarring to some extent. But even here, you would do well to experiment with a few lighter-weight foundations. The older you get, the less becoming are heavy products of any kind.

Though I don't recommend foundation for many mature skins, if you feel totally naked without it, at least try applying it a new way. Dampen a cosmetic sponge—you can buy them by the package in the cosmetic departments of most drugstores. These little sponges make many kinds of makeup go on more smoothly. Use the damp sponge to blend your foundation. Keep blending until you achieve the most natural look. Let the foundation dry, then proceed with your makeup. Take a good look at yourself, and I think you will agree that foundation looks best applied this way.

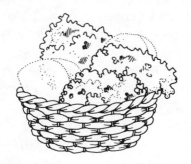

The other omission you may have noticed on the essentials list is lip gloss. Lip gloss just doesn't have the sophistication you need. It also tends to bleed into the tiny lines above your upper lip. A lipstick with real color and a nice creamy texture is a far better idea.

DRAWING THE PERFECT MOUTH

If you have been using lip gloss, now is the time to switch to a good clear lip color, a real lipstick. If you have been using lipstick, but you have been wearing deep, dramatic colors, think about changing to something lighter, something that isn't muddy or offbeat.

True clear reds, corals, tawny pinks, and peaches are all good colors for you. Pick a pink or peachy color, depending on what flatters your skin tone and eyes. Fair-skinned women with blue or hazel eyes look lovely in colors with a tawny pink overtone. Medium- to fair-skinned women with brown or even hazel eyes, look marvelous in colors with a coral or coral-brown tone. True brunette coloring can take the deepest lip colors, and clear reds look sensational on this coloring. Don't go overboard on deep colors; they look harsh even on brunettes.

If you have never used a *lip pencil,* do start to use one now. It will give much better definition to lips, especially if you have begun to develop tiny lines above your upper lip. Using a good lip pencil will keep the lip color from bleeding, because the texture of the pencil is firmer than a lipstick. There are two tricks to finding the right lip pencil. The first is finding the right texture. The pencil should not be too soft—it will be hard to work with and will bleed as badly as a lipstick—or too hard. What you want is a pencil that draws a clear, thin line without smudging or skipping. There are a great many pencils on the market, and many of them don't work well. Test before you buy. Make several lines on your hand to see that the pencil glides easily and doesn't skip; watch the tip, to see whether it tends to break off.

The second trick is finding the right color. This has little to do with your lipstick color, but everything to do with your lip color. A lip pencil's purpose is to give you a subtle, natural outline that will contain your lipstick. For this, the best color is a tawny, earthy color slightly darker than your natural lip color. Forget about matching or blending with your lipstick. Pink, red, and wine pencils always look artificial because the line never quite blends with the lipstick. An earth-colored pencil, on the other hand, blends into your lip color, giving the subtle, flattering illusion that just a bit of your natural lip line is showing around your lip color. The right lip-lining pencil can also help compensate for a too-thin, too-thick, or poorly shaped mouth.

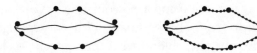

To use your lip pencil, look at the sketch. First, find the two little points, or tops, of your upper lip. Make a very subtle dot at each of the two points, then another dot at the low spot between the two points. Make two more tiny dots on your lower lip, exactly below the dots on the top lip. Make four more dots, at the corner, but not *in* the corner, of the top and bottom lips. Now connect the dots with lines, using a light hand with the pencil. If the line seems too dark, blot once gently with a tissue. Now apply lip color inside the dots. You should have a natural, soft-looking mouth. If your mouth is very thin, make all your dots and lines ever so slightly outside the natural lip line. If your lips are too full, make the dots just inside the lip line. If your mouth is crooked and one point on your upper lip is higher than the other, or your bottom lip is not quite straight, compensate by moving the dots slightly to "straighten" your lip line.

BLUSHING PERFECT CHEEKS

The most important thing I can tell you about blush is how it should be applied—and that is carefully. Too much and you look harsh, too little and you look washed out. I urge you not to be afraid of good, strong colors; they can be very flattering if applied correctly. The trick is to use one of two implements to apply the color. I prefer a sponge. There is nothing like it for blending. If you are using a powder blush, you can take up the color from the compact with the sponge and apply it directly, then blend with the opposite—clean—side of the sponge.

A flat or wedge-shaped sponge will work best. Use your fingers to apply cream blush, but blend with the sponge. A good sudsing once a week will remove accumulated color from the sponge. A brush, usually not the one that comes with your blusher, is also a good tool to use for application of powder blush. Go to the drugstore or an art-supply store and buy yourself a big, high-quality brush. The brushes that come with most blushers are too small and often flat. They don't make the best tool for getting a good application.

Take up some blush from the cake, tap the brush to remove excess powder, and apply color lightly to your cheeks. Stroke the brush across a tissue to remove powder and blend the color on your cheek with the brush again. Keep repeating this process until you have a nice glow on your cheek. Applying blusher correctly, getting both the amount of color you want and the correct placement, is tricky and takes practice, so plan to spend a little time perfecting your technique. You will be glad you did.

Now that you know how to apply blusher, the next question is *where* to apply it. Much has been written about how to contour your cheeks, but most of the advice does not work. Contouring to create hollows and high spots does work to some extent for photographic models, but for real people who are not going to be photographed for a fashion magazine, it is a waste of time. It almost always looks artificial and only looks good on someone who already has planes in her face—like a model. And if you look that good, you don't need to go to all that trouble. There are some things you can do, however, to give your face more interest.

First of all, you should always use blusher. It gives your face life and vitality. You have a choice between cream and powder; which you choose is largely a matter of personal taste. I think powder is easier to work with— you can blend it and make it look more subtle—but many women do admirably well with cream blushers. I would suggest you experiment with both. If you have always used one, try the other to see what you have been missing. Your skin texture and the amount of oil you produce has changed over the years, and you may find that a different type of blush works better now. If you have oily skin, a cream blush is not advisable, but if you have dry to normal skin, either will work.

You may have read that blush application should vary depending on your face shape. Actually, the most natural way to apply blush, no matter what your face shape, is in the little *kidney shape* you see in the sketch. You can vary this slightly, depending on face shape, but

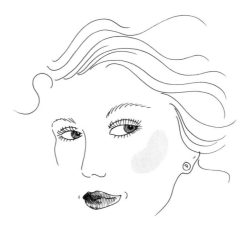

not much. If you have an oval face (considered to be the ideal face shape) or a squarish face (strong, prominent jawline), the top of the kidney should be on the top of your cheekbone, and the blush should blend into your hairline. If you have a long, slender face, slide the kidney down just a bit so that the top of it starts just under the cheekbone and extend the blusher into your hairline. This will give the illusion of a slightly broader face. If you have a round face, slide the kidney just a little closer to the center of your face and don't extend the blush all the way into your hairline. This will keep your face from appearing quite so round.

The one exception to my objection to contouring is the woman with strong, high cheekbones. Bones like this are a great beauty asset and you should make the most of them. Apply the blush in a kidney shape, high on your cheekbone. In the hollow under the bone, you might apply a very light amount of a deeper blush. Keep the two colors in the same tone, applying the lighter one on top and the deeper one in the cheek hollow. Blend well, so that you cannot see any demarcation line between the colors. Another attractive technique for highlighting this bone structure is done with a pearly powder or cream. Apply a very small amount of powder or cream on the bone, at the highest point of the cheekbone, and blend well. You want to create a small pool of light here to accent good bones.

YOUR BROWS, THE FRAME YOUR EYES NEED

Many a pretty eye has been spoiled by the wrong frame—the eyebrows. A well-shaped brow should start at the inside corner of your eyes and taper away gradually just beyond the outer corner. You should *always* follow the natural line of your brows. Don't force them into an artificial line. In general, it is better to tweeze stray hairs from below, rather than above the brow. You should always be certain the area between your brows is clean, with no straggly hairs. If you have good brows, all you need do is run an eyebrow brush over them when you have finished your makeup.

If your brows are sparse and droopy—and they probably are if you have fine hair—here are some good ideas that will help. Many women actually have brow hairs that are too long, and the end result is a brow line that droops because the hairs are long and fine. The solution: *Snip off the very ends of the hairs* with a pair of manicure scissors. Buy one of those little brow brushes with a tiny comb on one side. Comb up the hairs and snip off just the tips. Now brush through the brow. It will look more shapely and won't droop so much. You might also try using a little *mustache wax* or a light coat of mascara on your brows to help keep them in line.

If you want to darken your brows or fill in the gaps where hair is sparse, use either a well-sharpened brow pencil or one of those powder brow products made by many cosmetic companies. Either works well. Use a light hand with color, staying close to your own. Brows always look best when they are a shade or two *lighter* than your hair color.

WHAT BIG EYES YOU HAVE

Eyes are the trickiest features to make up. They have the potential to be tremendous beauty assets, but many women never tap that potential. Especially when you are forty or more, eyes are worth taking some time with. Because the tissue surrounding eyes is so delicate and not richly supplied with oil glands, this is one of the first areas to age. The upper lid stretches and becomes crinkly, making it a poor base for shadow, and the lower lid stretches and droops. Little bags and pouches also tend to form here. Before you read the chapter on cosmetic surgery, I would like to point out here that eye surgery is one of the most successful and simplest—for the patient—types of cosmetic surgery. It can also make the most dramatic difference in the way you look.

Since makeup techniques for eyes depend largely on how well the skin around your eyes has held up, I will give you two techniques. The first is for eyes that have begun to droop a bit, the second is for eyes that are in good shape.

FOR DROOPY EYES

If the skin over your upper eye is loose and crinkly, do *not* try to cover it with shadow. It will look terrible. You do want some color here, however. I suggest you buy yourself a couple of *good-quality eye pencils* and play with them. It pays to buy the best quality because the better the pencil the more smoothly it tends to go on and the less it tends to pull the skin as you apply it. A deep slate blue is pretty on blue eyes, a smoky, deep green is pretty on hazel eyes. Brown eyes are flattered by an earthy brown (one with a hint, but only a hint, of red) or a deep gray or a deep green, depending on what colors you are wearing close to your face.

Pick any of these colors that harmonize with a color you are wearing near your face. Now draw the pencil across your top lid, *close to the lash line.* Start at one corner and go all the way to the other. Smudge the line with your fingertip to soften it. Now, with the same pencil, make a line under your lower lid, close to the lash line, starting about the middle of your eye and extending to the outer corner. Smudge to soften the line. You can use your finger or a cotton-tipped swab to do this. The line should look soft and be very close to the lid. Finish your eye makeup with a couple of coats of mascara.

FOR EYES IN GOOD SHAPE

Even if the skin around your eyes is in good shape, do not go overboard with shadow. If you use too much, it will look harsh. Once again, buying a good-quality product is important because it will go on smoothly. Use either a powder or cream, but if you use a cream, check it several times during the day to see that it isn't creasing too much in the center of your lid. If it does, experiment with other brands of shadows; try a powder, too.

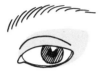

For an eye that has not begun to sag or crinkle, shadow applied in a soft wing looks marvelous.

If the skin around your eyes has begun to crinkle a bit, this makeup, concentrating shadow close to the lash line, is perfect.

You should stick to neutral, natural-looking colors like a soft brown, taupe, or gray shadow. Don't try pastels or dramatic colors such as burgundy or purples. They almost never look right on a mature woman. Using a good sponge-tipped applicator or a small brush for powder shadow and your finger for cream, apply shadow, starting at the inner corner of your eye. As you approach the outer corner, the arc of color should get wider and should slant *upward,* as it does in the sketch. The upward swing helps compensate for any droopiness. Now, staying very close to the bottom lashes, apply just a tiny bit of shadow under the lash, at the outer corner. If you're using cream shadow, don't use the cream on the lower lid. Instead, use a pencil in a shade as close to the shadow color as you can find and draw a soft line, smudging it to soften the look. Finish with the two coats of mascara, letting the first coat dry before applying the second.

This simple classic look—whether you choose the first or the second technique—is all you should apply for day. For evening, you can make the colors a bit more dramatic. Maybe try a small amount of gold or bronze powder dusted on lightly over the shadow or a dab of golden shadow smoothed on over your regular color to glaze it. You have to do a little experimenting before you find exactly the right look. The most important thing to remember is not to overdo. Too much of any kind of makeup makes you look harsh and has a tendency to be aging.

ACTION CHECKLIST FOR MAKEUP

- Reassess your face *now* and rethink your makeup in terms of your looks today.

- Decide what makeup essentials you need for your new look.

- Use cosmetic sponges to apply and blend blusher, foundation, and powder.

- Try a lip pencil.

- Learn where and how to apply blusher.

- Be objective about the condition of your eyes, and apply makeup accordingly.

MAKING UP WITH STYLE

WHAT THE EXPERTS SAY

Pablo Manzoni is a master at makeup. He is a witty, charming Italian from Florence who loves America, but also loves to point out that our puritanical heritage influences our ideas about life and looks. With his subtle Italian wit, he adores saying things that seem just a little bit outrageous to our American way of thinking.

Pablo has made up some of the most famous faces in the world, many of whom you may have seen in the pages of leading fashion magazines. After working for Elizabeth Arden for many years, he now has his own consulting business in New York City. Women come from all over the world for his famous makeup consultations. He has done wonderfully creative work on makeup after cosmetic surgery. It is essential, Pablo believes, to develop a new, updated look after any plastic surgery. His makeup wizardry is so successful, however, that he often helps a woman avoid surgery by showing her how to look younger with makeup. Here are some of Pablo's ideas about makeup.

What is your attitude about beauty and midlife?

So many women have preconceived notions about their looks. They can become not so much unattractive as dated. That's when it's time to change. Middle age is an American invention. A woman in her forties is "borderline" in America. Italian, French, and Spanish have no direct translation for "middle age." It is unfortunate that, since Americans seem to like all things continental, they haven't also adopted the continental at-

titude about women. A woman at midlife is so much more interesting, so seasoned, so much better to talk to and be around
than a very young woman.

What do women most often do wrong with their makeup and looks?

Too often, women try to correct their features with makeup,
and it always shows. Hollywood is partly responsible for this
because it presents such plastic, ideal beauties for us to imitate.
It's far better to play up a good feature than to hide a bad or
aging one. Exaggeration is another big mistake. Too much of
anything looks wrong. There's no need to wear everything you
have on your dressing table at one time. An exaggerated
makeup is a mask to hide behind.

What helps a woman look young?

Short hair is rejuvenating. Making the hair a little bit lighter is
also a help. Your object should also be hair that looks as if you
can run your fingers through it. Many mature women make the
mistake of being too "coiffed." A woman should also learn to
develop her own style. She needs to understand that just because
something is in fashion doesn't mean it's right for her. By the
time you've reached forty, you should have a sure sense of what
works for you. This can keep you looking well for the rest of
your life.

What kind of makeup is most flattering?

A well-blended rouge is one of your best makeup assets. It looks
young and alive. Avoid powder, except on your nose, and avoid
heavy foundations. No foundation or a very light water-based
one, or a tinted moisturizer, are best for mature skins. A dark

"perky" eye is also a tremendous asset. Eyes are commanding, and they should be well made up. Neutral shadows—brown, gray, or plum—are the best choices. You can be daring if you use these good neutrals. When a woman looks down, she should never have a slab of turquoise going across her lids! Smoky colors, well blended, look much prettier from any angle.

Have you any suggestions for correcting shadows or circles?

You will deemphasize under-eye problems by bringing your rouge up as high on your cheeks as possible. Bring it up almost under the eye. If it is blended well, it looks like a neutral, healthy flush. Remember to keep your brows as light as possible. Never darken them unless they are very pale. Also, try to make them appear as high as possible. Use a very deep, well-blended neutral shadow on the lid and a lighter tone of the same color under the brow, bringing it down to meet the darker shadow. Never wear pale highlighters under your brow. A deep color makes the brows look higher and more youthful. A darker color under the brow gives the eye wonderful depth. Don't forget you have two lids. Bring your shadow under the lower lid and blend it well.

Today, glasses can be a wonderful makeup item. Many beautiful women wear them as an accessory, not because they really need them. Tinted lenses can make eyes look lovely. The only caution here is to be sure the top of your frame comes up to your eyebrow. If your brows show above the frames, you have two lines there—your brow and the glass frame—which is unattractive.

What finishing touches do you suggest?

I always advise my clients to get dressed and made up, then stand in front of a full-length mirror and see what they can do without. Can you remove some jewelry for a simpler, more elegant look? Could you do with a little less makeup? Should it be blended a bit more here or there? And, finally, don't worry about little flaws. A perfect face is not memorable, but a face with some small flaw often is!

C H A P T E R 6

M I D L I F E

W O M E N A N D

S U C C E S S

How successful can you be at midlife? What do you have to look forward to? To help you answer these questions, consider the unique achievements of some very successful midlife women—an actress, a musical-comedy star, a model, and a businesswoman. The women you are going to read about are at the peak of their success, with as much to look forward to as they have to look back on. Life, for them, continues to promise nearly unending possibilities for the future. These women have not been discouraged by the clock—and you don't have to be either. Read about them and be inspired.

KAREN BLACK, ACTRESS

Karen Black has no fear of forty. She not only hopes to have another child in addition to her son, Hunter, but she also sees her career in films expanding continuously. Karen, who recently starred in both the off-Broadway play and the movie, *Come Back to the Five and Dime, Jimmy Dean, Jimmy Dean*, soared into fame with her performance opposite Jack Nicholson in *Five Easy Pieces*. Since then, she has appeared in many movies, including *The Great Gatsby, Easy Rider, Nashville, Portnoy's Complaint, Family Plot, Burnt Offerings, Day of the Locust*, and *Can She Bake a Cherry Pie?*

Karen does not deny that forty is a watershed age for a woman. "I have some ambivalence," she says, "but basically, I have a concept of life as being very long. I don't feel limited by time or life. I'm a creative person and I'll get into other areas of film as well as acting."

Good looks are a tremendous asset in the movies, but, says Karen, "I don't feel you can go very far in Hollywood as just another pretty face. The really interesting parts are character parts." Though she does not feel that growing older has to hamper a woman, she does admit to occasional anger. "I see a wrinkle and I think, if I were a man, if I were Paul Newman, it wouldn't matter how old I am or how many wrinkles I get. Men age and women can't is still part of some people's value system. But," she goes on, "I don't feel this way very often. I think the reality is getting too obvious to miss. Women can't be put down or cast aside because they pass forty. Also, I think women of forty today look ten years younger than women of forty did a generation ago. Women of fifty and older look years younger than

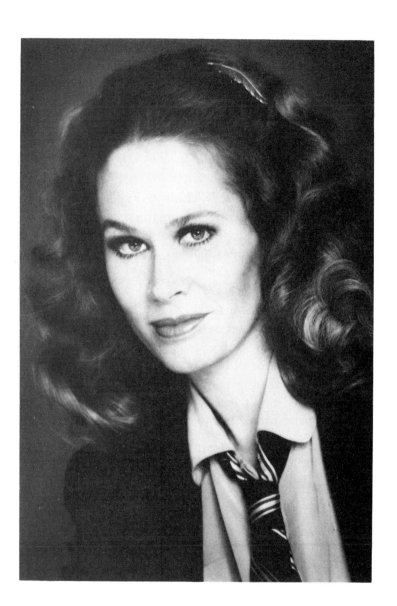

women used to look at that age. Women are having babies later, too. Doctors no longer get hysterical when a forty-year-old woman wants to have a baby. The curve of a woman's life is changing and lengthening. I still want to have another baby."

When Karen talks about her career now, she says, "Your product becomes better and better because you've got more to give as you age. This is an innate attitude for me. Interest in life is what keeps you young. Failed purposes give you more of a sense of age than years. Women must learn that if they fail in one area, there are many others they can succeed in. You mustn't carry around a sense of failed purposes."

When she talks about her looks, Karen says she does not believe in dieting, but in eating correctly. "The roller coaster of dieting, of eating a lot then a little, is so bad for your body." Karen has her own unique view of how she should eat, and, clearly, it works well for her. "I like to eat the whole of something," she says. "I'll eat a whole potato or a whole cabbage and call it a meal. Also, if I eat something fried in a day, I make it a point not to eat something sweet. I don't like to mix raw and cooked foods. I'll eat whatever is raw—a salad, for example—then eat the cooked foods. I like to eat a complex carbohydrate for breakfast, because it stays with me, gives me energy for many hours."

Karen's view of exercise is as unique as her attitudes about food. "I think exercise should be a way to give your body attention. I like to concentrate on the parts of my body that have a problem. If my shoulders are feeling tense, I'll concentrate exercise on them. I think your body talks to you, tells you where it needs attention. I like to give my body peaceful attention. Yoga exercises are a wonderful way to do this. They stretch your body slowly to keep you fluid and flexible. Paying attention to your body is a healing process. If you listen to your body and pay attention to it, it will respond positively. If you aren't in tune with yourself, you can create problems, cause tension and stress."

Karen's philosophy obviously works for her. She has never looked more beautiful, never felt better about herself nor had more confidence in her future. She is in one of the most fickle and difficult businesses for a woman, and her attitude is undoubtedly what will continue to keep her on top. The same kind of positive attitude can make any woman more successful.

KAYLAN PICKFORD, MODEL

Kaylan Pickford is a study in courage and determination. She began to model at forty-five, an age when most models have long since stepped away from the camera. In a field where youth is supreme, where the average age of a model keeps going down, rather than up, she's defied the rules.

Kaylan, a New Englander by birth and temperament, lived in California and Washington, D.C., before coming to New York. "I needed the energy of New York," she says. Only a few months after a new marriage, she moved from California to Washington, where her husband became terminally ill with cancer. Four difficult years later, he died. Kaylan had never worked and had no real skills. Courageously, she came to New York. She started modeling by accident. An agent asked if she modeled, and she could tell from the way he asked the

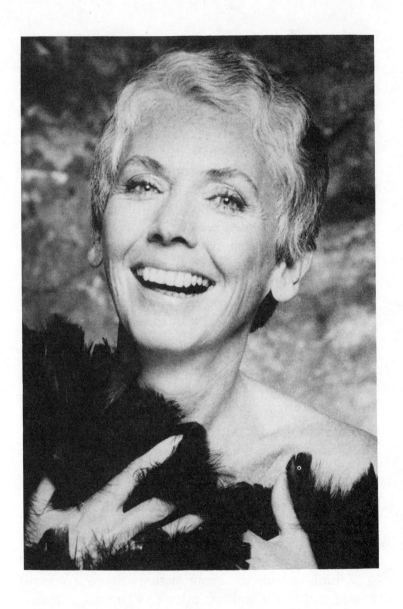

question that he assumed she did. "I just let him keep on assuming," she says, "and I got my first job. Sex sells products, and in our society, sex equals youth," so jobs at first were hard to come by. "I just hung in and, little by little, it began to click."

Today, you can see Kaylan's beautiful face and her trademark short, silvery hair on television and in magazines everywhere. Talking with her, you immediately sense her professionalism—a great asset in a field populated by young, inexperienced girls—and her serenity. For Kaylan, life has not been easy. Living through tragedy, enduring hardships have given her a sense of herself as a survivor that many women never achieve.

After modeling for a few years, Kaylan decided to write a book about her experiences because she wanted to inspire other women. "I wanted them to see that at forty-five or fifty and beyond, there could be beauty, sexuality, the works." The glowing array of photographs of her in *Always a Woman* prove her point better than any words could.

Today Kaylan is a successful top model. "I can tell immediately when I go to a job whether the people there know what they're doing. If the art director is a twelve-year-old, I know there'll be trouble. To be truly creative, you have to have some seasoning. When advertising was so hooked on youth and young people, they took all the creativeness out of it. Things were done for their shock value or because they were attention-getting, but they weren't truly creative. Now we've begun to swing back.

"I think our attitude about mature women has come a long way but it still has a long way to go." Kaylan hopes that women like her will make it easier for others to feel good about themselves. "The key is what's going on in your head," she says, "how you see yourself." She feels that a woman radiates good things if she feels good about herself. "If you don't feel good about you, no one else will! Using yourself is the best thing. If you don't use your creative juices, you aren't living." Why has she been successful when other models her age are out of the business? "It's worked for me because I'm saying something positive about myself, I'm saying that there's life, beauty, and hope after forty."

GILLIS MACGILL, BUSINESSWOMAN, FORMER MODEL

Gillis MacGill has the best of all worlds. For years, she was a celebrated model wearing the clothes of every famous designer in New York as well as the big names in European fashion. Then she turned modeling into a profitable business by starting Mannequin, a model agency for fashion-show models. Gillis currently runs the agency and acts as spokeswoman for the Celanese Corporation.

Gillis loved modeling, but, she says, "Today it's running the business that gives me my chief satisfaction. There were times when I considered giving it up because I was so busy, but I didn't and I'm so grateful now."

Gillis says she always wanted to be a model, from the moment "I realized it was the perfect thing to do with my tall, skinny body. I couldn't believe I could make a career out of what I'd been so embarrassed about as a teen-ager." Gillis did have the perfect body for modeling—and the perfect face, strong with wonderful, high

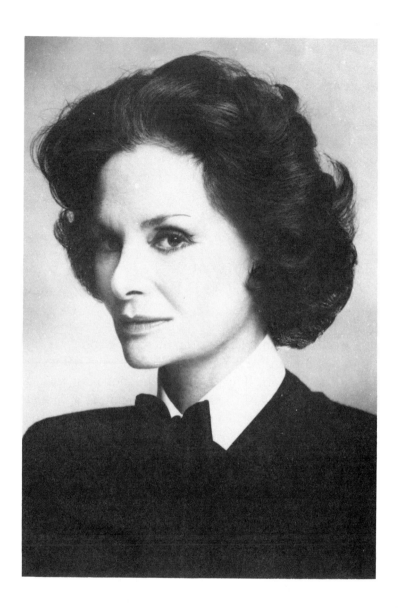

cheekbones framed by glossy dark hair. She was a great success and, she says, "I never thought about whether I'd be forced to stop modeling one day. Then, when I was thirty, a friend said, 'Gillis, you're at your peak now.' I thought, God, if I'm at my peak now, there's only one way to go and that's down. I was shocked. It was just about this time that the idea of a modeling business came to me. There were about five of us at Plaza 5 {a well-known agency} who did a lot of fashion shows. We realized that booking a model for a fashion show was a lot different from booking one for a photographic sitting. A friend suggested that we start an agency just for fashion-show models and that I run it. At first, the idea seemed crazy, but the more I thought about it, the more sense it made—and that's how Mannequin was born.

"I sympathize with today's young women who want to do it all, have it all. I was the same way, and there were times when being a wife, mother, model, and businesswoman were more than I could handle. I thought of giving up the agency, but today it's the thing that sustains me, keeps me active and alive. When I look back, I realize I never believed I'd get to be forty. Oh, no, it couldn't happen to me—then it did, and unbelievably fast. I never believed I'd reach the point when my twin sons wouldn't need constant attention. They grew up, of course, and I can't believe how quickly. Even though you sometimes feel you can't handle any more, I think it's important to do as much as you can. You never know just how much you can do until you try. You must be constantly testing your limits. I've discovered that I am the kind of person who has great difficulty doing just a little. I have to do nothing at all—take a day for myself to indulge in whatever I like—or I have to be truly, creatively busy.

"I think aging, like most things, has its benefits. One of the benefits is learning what gives you pleasure. You discover, as you grow older, what you like and what you don't. When you're very young, you're too busy getting ahead to take the time to know much about yourself. As you age, you begin to learn who you are. When I look at my life now, I feel the easiest part is behind me, but that doesn't necessarily mean I'm not excited about what's ahead. I remember my mother saying to me when I was young, 'If I could only put my head on your shoulders.' I know what she meant now. Now, at least, I think I have some of the wisdom my mother was talking about and I intend to use it well.

"I feel there's no denying we're still a youth-oriented society. I don't like to say it, but it's true. It has changed a bit, and it continues to change, but it hasn't changed enough. I do know, happily, that my sons' attitudes are very different from mine at their age, and I'm glad.

"I feel very optimistic about my life now because I know I am a creative and competent person. One of the greatest things I've learned is that the skills I may not have myself are available to me through other people. I no longer feel frustrated if I can't do something myself. I don't have to do it all anymore; in fact, I've learned it's not desirable to do it all. We all have a support system for achieving our goals and we must learn to use it. The women's movement can be an important support system for every woman.

"As I've gotten older, I've become easier on myself. I'm also easier on the people I work with. Aging is a mellowing process. We become more self-accepting, less self-doubting—and this alone makes it all worthwhile!"

LILIANE MONTEVECCHI,
MUSICAL·COMEDY STAR

Liliane Montevecchi is vintage champagne. Her success is golden, her enthusiasm for life effervescent. French by birth, Ms. Montevecchi has been a star both here and in Europe. Her sense of discipline and dedication come from ballet training. She was prima ballerina in Roland Petit's famous French company, starred in the Folies-Bergère, and has also appeared in many American movies, including *Daddy Long Legs*, in which she danced with Fred Astaire. Most recently Ms. Montevecchi won a Tony award for her performance in the smash-hit Broadway musical *Nine*.

You would have to go a long way to find a woman with a more positive attitude about life than Liliane Montevecchi. "I don't give getting old a thought," she says. "I only think how good I feel. I make it a practice never to want things I know I can't have. I can walk down the street and see a beautiful jewel in a shop window and admire it, but I never feel unhappy about not being able to have it. I feel this way about all aspects of my life. Don't make yourself unhappy about what you can't have—including youth.

"I am successful and privileged now, but if success goes, I can handle it. I can ride in a limo or the bus and be happy. If I ride the bus, I amuse myself thinking about what all the people do—where do they work, who

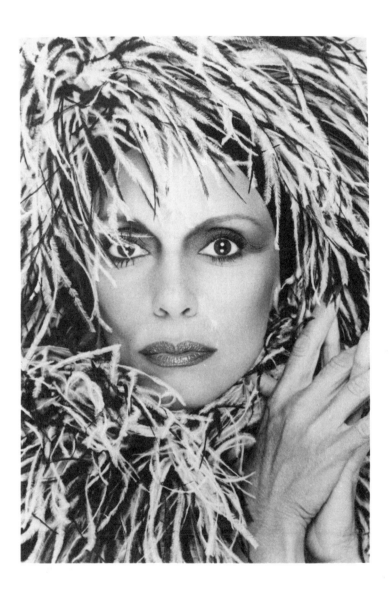

are they married to, what did they eat for breakfast. To me, life is a continual amusement.

"I get more attention from men now than I ever did. I don't do anything in particular to get it, it just comes to me and I enjoy it."

Like many midlife women, Ms. Montevecchi considers work very important. "I can't imagine not working. I'd like to do a play soon. I know I can't do a formal ballet anymore—I'm too old—but I will always dance, if it's in the context of a play." Work, she feels, is restorative. She has no particular plans for what she'll do next. "I'm like a cork in the sea," she says. "Wherever the waves take me, I'll go."

Ms. Montevecchi also shares another attitude with midlife women. "I've learned so many things that now I'd like to begin giving back to others some of what I've learned. When I was young, I surrounded myself with older people to 'water my plant,' so to speak. Now I'd like to water someone else's plant. Younger women have more attractive bodies, but older women have more experience to give, and that's terribly important."

Growth is something many women are preoccupied with at midlife. "As you get older, your energy goes to other things," she says, "but you must still grow. You must experience things, so you have no regrets when you are really old. Generally, we regret the things we didn't do, not the ones we did!"

Ms. Montevecchi credits her incredible figure to many hours of dance practice a week and to "eating only when I'm hungry. Some days," she says, "I don't eat anything until three in the afternoon, because I'm not hungry." Then she adds with a mischievous wink: "Clams, I love clams and they don't have many calories." She doesn't worry much about her looks. "People are very accepting of me, so I know everything must look pretty good," she laughs. And everything does look good, from her sleek dark hair to her broad smile—which she flashes frequently—to her beautiful, slender, expressive hands—the hands of a dancer.

"People don't want to be bored by anyone, you need to keep yourself interesting," she says, and it's a pretty safe bet that this enthusiastic, ageless beauty will never bore anyone!

CHAPTER 7

COSMETIC SURGERY — BIG COMMITMENT, BIG DIVIDENDS

No woman should make the decision to have cosmetic surgery without serious consideration and a totally realistic attitude. Deciding to undergo surgery involves more commitment than any other beauty procedure, but the dividends it can pay are large. Cosmetic surgery *is* surgery, and, though the risks are minimal, no surgery is completely risk-free. Another consideration: The changes made are permanent. Once done, you cannot undo the results. Therefore, it is imperative that you give any procedure careful consideration and know exactly what to expect.

IS IT BAD TO WANT SOMETHING GOOD?

Americans have a puritanical heritage. Though this heritage has provided us with many benefits, such as a strong work ethic, it has also given us more than a few problems. Trouble in the bedroom can often be traced directly to a puritanical point of view. Less serious, but just as directly related to our past, were our notions of only a few decades ago that any woman who painted her fingernails or colored her hair was "bad." Few people entertain such judgmental and moralistic attitudes about these innocent things today, though hair coloring is still tainted with a bit of this kind of thinking.

Cosmetic surgery is probably the last holdover in this area. A great many men and women wrestle with a puritanical feeling about surgery. This feeling is behind their desire to keep secret the fact that they have had surgery. It is surprising, indeed, that in this age of self-improvement and fitness, anyone still harbors such ideas about cosmetic surgery.

A specific complaint lodged against cosmetic surgery is that it is just plain frivolous. But why shouldn't we want to look our best? Attitudes have come a long way in recent years, and, surprisingly enough, the government has been a leader. Cosmetic surgery is now a tax-deductible expense and has been for several years.

Certainly surgery is a more serious business than painting your nails or coloring your hair, but the same rationale lies behind it—or going on a diet, or learning how to use makeup properly, or going to a therapist. You want to make yourself look better, feel better, and function better. Is there anything wrong with that? Clearly not, and more and more people are realizing it. Increasing numbers of respected, intelligent women are stepping forward, proud to announce that they have had surgery. They regard it as a responsibility to themselves to stay at their best. Bravo!

WHY CONSIDER SURGERY?

Since at least the time of Aristotle, it has been common to make assumptions about people based on looks. Aristotle wrote that men with small foreheads were fickle, that straight eyebrows indicated softness of disposition, and that large ears indicated a tendency to talk too much. Fortunately, we don't believe these things today, but it is surprising how much we do assume about people based on looks. One of the best examples of how we judge people by a physical feature is the man or woman with aging eyelids. Drooping upper lids and bags under the eyes make you look tired, even when you may be feeling energetic. Anyone who wants to be seen as vital and alive has something basic to overcome if she has tired-looking eyes. As you age, your face tends to sag and the contours, once tight and sleek, tend to droop. This droopiness can make you look tired and lackluster. One of the main reasons for cosmetic surgery is to correct this false impression. In addition to a tired look, drooping facial contours make people believe you are older than you are. If this is translated into a prejudice about your ability to do your job, it can be unfortunate. Correcting all these false impressions is a valid reason to have cosmetic surgery.

There is also one other good reason—your own unhappiness with your appearance. Yvonne, at forty-five, was a lively, vital woman deeply engrossed in community activities after raising her children. She looked at a picture of herself in the local paper, taken at a community fund-raising event, and was shocked by what she saw. She looked ten years older than she felt. The vitality that surged inside her did not seem evident on her face. In short, she was deeply unhappy with the way she looked. She did not want to look twenty-five again, but she did want to look as good as she felt. Yvonne decided to have cosmetic surgery.

WHEN IS SURGERY A MISTAKE?

Though cosmetic surgery can do astonishing things, it cannot work miracles, as one unhappy woman learned. Mary was forty-five and desperately unhappy. She suspected that her husband was having an affair with another woman and, distraught over this, she had been unable to work constructively at her job. Her boss and co-workers noticed her drop in productivity. Her husband sensed her unhappiness. Mary was also unhappy about her appearance. Always thought of as a beauty, she felt that she had lost her looks and associated all her problems with this loss.

She finally decided to see a plastic surgeon for a consultation. She poured out her troubles to the doctor and ended by saying that she felt sure her life would improve after surgery. Wisely, the doctor told her in the gentlest way he could that he did not feel she would be a good candidate for surgery. Then Mary went to another surgeon who was not quite so ethical. This surgeon agreed to perform a face lift. The surgery, by all normal standards, was a complete success, but Mary regarded it as a dismal failure. Her husband finally left her, and her problems at work became worse than ever.

Mary had unrealistic expectations. She believed that a change in her looks would make her husband love her again and would restore her old energy on the job. Since her real problems had nothing to do with her appearance, changing her looks did not change her problems. The first surgeon was wise enough to realize this.

Cosmetic surgery can make a significant difference in the way you look, but it will not solve emotional problems. However, a face lift or eye lift can make you feel more comfortable with your looks, can take away that tired, drawn look, and these benefits can help you be a more productive, appealing human being. If you don't expect miracles, just a nice little ego boost, you're on the right track.

If you look in the mirror and see bags under your eyes or loose skin at your chin line, you may feel certain that you would love seeing these imperfections disappear. Once they do disappear, however, you may feel different. You did not become middle-aged overnight, but you *will* lose the loose, slack look overnight, and sometimes this can be hard to accept. Even though you are not happy with the face you see, you have been seeing it for a great many years and any substantial change can be unsettling. After cosmetic surgery, a woman may look at her face and wonder if the skin around her eyes looks too tight or whether the inevitable tiny scars are too noticeable. She may wonder if the surgeon made both sides of her face symmetrical or if the line on one side of her mouth is deeper than the one on the other. Many women experience depression after cosmetic surgery similar to the postpartum blues some women experience after having a baby. Just as producing a lovely, healthy baby may not seem as momentous as you had thought, getting rid of lines and wrinkles may not provide the high you expected. If your expectations are realistic, however, you will quickly get beyond this period and emerge happy and confident with your new look.

WHAT CAN SURGERY DO?

Basically, cosmetic surgery *removes excess skin* so that the contours of your face look smoother and sleeker. It does not necessarily remove wrinkles. In some cases, when the skin is stretched more tightly over your bone and muscle structure, wrinkles do appear less noticeable, but, by and large, cosmetic surgery is not a wrinkle eraser. It is a loose-skin remover.

Crow's-feet, frown lines, horizontal lines in the forehead, lines around your mouth are not usually removed as the result of a face lift, but there are ways to make these lines less noticeable, and I will discuss them later in this chapter.

FINDING THE RIGHT SURGEON

Finding the right surgeon is more than just finding somebody competent. You want a doctor you feel a connection to, a rapport with. In order to find this person, you are probably going to have to talk to several surgeons. As with any surgery, you would be wise to have more than one consultation. You need not feel embarrassed if you do not sign up upon leaving the office. You may not feel this is the right surgeon, or you may feel you cannot afford a surgeon, or you may simply feel you are not yet ready to have surgery. Any or all of these feelings are quite normal.

When you first visit a surgeon, get a feel for his or her approach to your problems. Try to discover whether the doctor is sympathetic to your needs, whether he or she inspires confidence. You should make *a list of questions* to ask before you go, so you won't forget anything while you are there. You will probably want to see one or more surgeons in addition to the first one. It is usually a good idea to see at least two doctors before making any decision. There are many surgical approaches to any particular operation and you may feel more comfortable with one rather than another. For example, some surgeons prefer to do all their operating under general anesthesia. Others use local anesthesia for all but the most complicated procedures. Either approach is considered correct, but you may have a preference for one and you won't get a clear picture of what your options are unless you talk to more than one doctor. You will also find that some procedures, such as eye lifts, can be done on an outpatient basis, which may be desirable if you have a fear of hospitals. Cosmetic surgery is neither simple nor cheap. Ask questions, gather your options, then decide.

Getting the names of several surgeons should not be difficult. *Word of mouth* is one of the best sources of information. A friend who has had a successful experience with a surgeon is often the finest recommendation you can get. If this method doesn't work, ask your family doctor or your gynecologist to give you a couple of names. Your county and state medical societies can also supply you with names. You should always be certain that any doctor you consider is *board certified* to practice cosmetic surgery. There are doctors who do such operations but are not certified by the board of cosmetic surgeons. It is not a good idea to go to such a doctor. Cosmetic surgery is a delicate, highly demanding kind of surgery, and you can be certain of the results only if you choose a doctor who specializes in and is certified in this type of surgery.

Consultation fees and how they are billed vary widely. Some doctors charge a flat fee for consultation, payable at your appointment. Others charge a fee if you decide not to have surgery, but include the fee in the cost of surgery if you do go ahead. You should ask what the fee involves when you make your appointment. You may be surprised to learn that the surgical fee for a cosmetic operation almost always is paid in advance. This is done because many patients cancel surgery at the last minute; a requirement of payment in advance helps a surgeon separate the serious patients from those who will not follow through. If he scheduled time in the operating room of a hospital and you canceled, he would be in trouble, but if you have paid in advance, he knows you are serious about the surgery. There are also women whose expectations about the surgery are so unrealistic that they would never pay afterward—because these expectations could never be met. If the surgeon does a competent job, he is entitled to his fee. It is not his fault if all your problems are not solved by the surgery.

TAKING PICTURES

Do not be surprised if your surgeon directs you to a special photographer to have preoperative photographs of your face taken. These photographs, usually taken while you are wearing no makeup, will be used as a guide in surgery. Because of the anesthesia and the fact that you are lying down during surgery, your face is not in its normal state. The pictures help the surgeon know how much correction is needed. Many surgeons request postoperative photographs as well. These are kept in his file for comparison in case you want further surgery in the future.

BLEPHAROPLASTY OR EYE-LIFT SURGERY

Of all cosmetic procedures, this one can produce the most dramatic results. It is also one of the quickest and easiest cosmetic procedures to recover from. From thirty-five on, the delicate skin around your eyes begins to show some of the effects of aging. The upper eyelids can sag and become "crepey." The little fat pouches under your eyes can push forward, causing under-eye bags. Some puffiness, as a result of heredity, can appear as early as the mid- and late twenties. These bags can be quite unattractive and make an otherwise vital face look old and tired. Removal of the bags produces dramatic results.

It is becoming increasingly common for cosmetic surgeons to do certain procedures in their offices. For this they may set up *in-office operating rooms* or they may have private facilities in an office setting that they share with several other surgeons. Eyelid surgery is one of the operations that is commonly done in the office. The theory behind this is that the patient does not need to take up a hospital bed nor does she have to be subjected to the unpleasantness and expense of a hospital stay. The eyelid-lift procedure takes only about two to two and a half hours and is relatively uncomplicated, though quite delicate. If the operation is done in an office setting, the patient is usually heavily sedated, but not put under general anesthesia. After surgery, the patient rests in the doctor's office until she has recovered enough to go home, usually several hours later.

The actual operation involves making two incisions, the first in the top lid, normally about halfway between the eyelashes and the eyebrow. Excess skin is trimmed away and the incision is stitched closed. A second incision is made under the lower lashes and, once again, loose skin is trimmed away. If the fatty pads here have protruded to form bags, some of the fatty deposit is removed. The incision is then closed. Both incisions are concealed in natural folds of the eyes so that visible scarring is minimal. There will be some scars, as it is impossible to cut skin without leaving scar tissue.

Most patients can resume normal life after about two weeks. You will have considerable swelling and discoloration for the first few days, but there is usually little if any discomfort following an eye lift. Ice compresses are applied for the first day after surgery to reduce swelling and control bruising. Pain, if there is any, can be relieved with a mild painkiller and usually subsides completely within twenty-four hours. You then feel nothing but a little tightness. Depending on your surgeon's technique, stitches are removed three to five days later. After about two weeks, most of the swelling and redness will disappear. The incision lines may remain pink for several months but a little makeup conceals this. The results of an eye lift are enduring, usually as much as ten or more years. Under-eye bags seldom return, though tissue may stretch and sag, necessitating another operation ten to fifteen years later.

QUESTIONS TO ASK YOUR DOCTOR ABOUT AN EYE LIFT

What kind of anesthesia will you use?

Will the operation be done in a hospital or an office?

If the procedure is done in a hospital, how long will I have to stay?

What are your fees?

What will hospitalization cover?

When will the stitches come out?

When can I wash my hair? Color it?

When will I be able to wear eye makeup?

When can I wear contact lenses?

When can I return to work or social activities?

What complications can I expect based on my health and the condition of my eyes?

How long will the results last in my case?

Should I avoid the sun? For how long?

FACE LIFT OR
RHYTIDECTOMY

A total face lift includes an eye lift, but the two procedures need not be done at the same time. Very often, the eyes need help before the face does. In such a case, the eye lift is performed first, with a face lift to follow several years later. Though not as delicate a surgical procedure as an eye lift, a face lift is more complicated because it involves more incisions, thus disturbing more nerves and blood vessels. It also takes longer. Many surgeons still prefer to do a face lift under general anesthesia, though the trend is away from a general because it involves slightly more risks. Most face lifts are performed in a hospital or hospitallike setting, but this too is changing as more and more plastic surgeons acquire in-office operating-room facilities.

There are many approaches to a face lift, but the most common involves making an incision in the hairline at the temples. The incision continues down in front of and around the ear. The excess skin is trimmed away and the incision closed. A second incision is made in the hairline on the back of the head, just behind the ear. This gives the chin and neck a nice, smooth line. Although there are many variations to this procedure, it is the basic one followed by most surgeons.

Some surgeons bring the incision down into the ear itself so that there will be no visible incision line on the face. This procedure can sometimes result in a rather clumsy looking earlobe. When the incision is made just in front of the ear, there is a tiny scar, but it falls into a natural skin fold and is almost invisible. A good surgeon can close the incision so that the scarring is imperceptible. The in-the-ear procedure seems something of a gimmick used by surgeons to convince prospective patients that they are better than other surgeons. Your decision on who is best for you should be made on more solid information than this.

The face-lift operation usually lasts several hours, and takes longer if the eyes are being done at the same time. When you wake up, you will find your head swathed in bandages to minimize swelling. The bandages come off within seventy-two hours, usually sooner, and no new ones need be applied. The visible stitches are usually removed on about the fifth day. Those in the hairline are removed on the tenth day or thereabouts. Stitches that are in an area that will show are removed first to minimize scarring. The others are left in longer because there is more pressure on these incision lines.

You will be quite swollen as well as black and blue for some time after surgery. Most of the visible swelling and discoloration will disappear in about two weeks, but you will remain swollen for several months, though you may not be aware of it. You can also expect some pain and discomfort, especially for the first forty-eight hours. Make certain your doctor leaves instructions for painkillers, so that you do not have to suffer while a nurse tries to reach him for permission to give you medication. Most doctors do this routinely, but it is always a good idea to double-check.

In addition to some pain, you should be prepared to experience feelings of numbness in your ears and cheeks. This occurs because many of the small facial nerves have been disturbed during surgery. Most of the feeling will return, but it can take several months. Some patients experience a great deal of numbness in their ears, especially. One woman explained it this way, "I felt as though my ears were fragile china plates that would break if touched. It was a very strange feeling." Just how much discomfort you experience as a result of the whole procedure depends on your pain tolerance, your surgeon, and on your degree of apprehension. The more nervous you are, the more discomfort you are likely to feel. This is a very good reason to find a surgeon you trust and to get as much information beforehand as you can. The entire procedure will go more smoothly if you do.

One additional complication you may experience is *mild hair loss*. Most doctors won't tell you about this because they consider it routine and inconsequential. To a woman who does not expect it, it can seem anything but inconsequential. Hair loss is usually in the temple areas. The surgeon makes his incision deep enough to get below the germinating portion of the hair, but, depending on your hair's reaction to trauma, some of the roots may die. This loss is usually not permanent, but it can be unnerving to see hair coming out on your comb several weeks after surgery. Some women are so alarmed that they fear they are going bald. While most of the hair that comes out will regrow, it is possible that some won't. You are also likely to experience some slight hair loss in the back of your head around the incisions. One woman experienced a great deal of loss. "I had two distinct round bald spots in the back of my head. I was horrified and felt I had made a poor trade—baldness in return for a smooth face. Later, I learned that the spots were caused because of lowered blood pressure during surgery and then continued pressure on the spots from lying in bed for a week afterward. The hair grew back, but it took six months and I couldn't find anyone who could explain what had happened. Finally, my dermatologist explained it: he told me it's not uncommon in any kind of surgery when blood pressure is lowered. Reducing the blood supply to hair roots and lying on your back for some time can cause temporary hair loss on the pressure points on the back of your head." Although this woman's experience was extreme, some variation can and often does occur. Usually it is not a problem so long as you realize that most of the hair will regrow.

Your surgeon may also shave a patch of hair away at the temple to make working there easier. This is not absolutely necessary. Many surgeons do not shave because they realize it makes it difficult to style the hair for as much as six months afterward. This is something you should discuss with your doctor. If he is a shaver, you may want to ask him to make an exception or even find a doctor who feels it is not necessary. Men's hair is not shaved for a face lift because it would be too noticeable, so why should you have to put up with having yours shaved!

A properly done face lift will make you look relaxed and rested and in many cases can make you look as much as ten years younger. The results can be expected to last about ten years. You must remember that you continue to age from the minute you have your face lift, but you will always look younger than your chronological age.

Technically speaking, an eye lift and a face lift are the two operations that correct facial aging. But many people are motivated by age to have cosmetic surgery and

QUESTIONS TO ASK YOUR DOCTOR ABOUT A FACE LIFT

What kind of anesthesia will you use?

Where will the surgery be done, in your office or in a hospital?

How long will I be hospitalized?

What are your fees?

What will my hospitalization cover?

What results can I expect from surgery?

When will the stitches come out?

Do you shave hair? Where, how much?

When will I be able to wash my hair?

When can I have it colored?

When can I wear makeup?

When will I be able to go back to work or be seen socially?

What complications can I expect?

How long will results last for me?

Should I avoid the sun? For how long?

decide that once they are going to have surgery, they might as well have some other corrections made. For example, Linda decided to have an eye lift and felt that as long as she was going to undergo surgery, she would have her nose operated on, too. For years, she had hated its long aquiline shape and she decided that she would change that as well as get rid of the bags under her eyes. Linda's doctor told her she had made the right decision because, as we age, our noses drop and get slightly longer. Usually this is not noticeable, but in Linda's case, since she was unhappy with her nose to begin with, time would only make her more unhappy.

Margaret decided it was time for a face lift and she discussed with her doctor the possibility of a chin implant as well. The doctor explained that he could easily insert a silicone implant in Margaret's receding chin to give it a better line. Deciding to combine procedures as these women did is not uncommon. Just because you have lived with something for forty years does not mean you have to live with it for another forty.

NOSE RECONSTRUCTION OR RHINOPLASTY

Nose reconstruction can accomplish dramatic changes. A bump in the bridge can be smoothed out, a too-long nose can be shortened, a crooked nose can be straightened. Fixing wide, flaring nostrils is less successful, but sometimes possible. You must discuss with your surgeon exactly what you want done to find out if it is feasible. One of the chief difficulties with nose surgery is that you are permanently changing a feature. If you have an eye lift or a face lift, you are simply making your face look younger and more rested, more the way it used to look. You are not really altering your appearance radically. Creating a "new" feature is something you must be well prepared for. It is important that you discuss with your doctor exactly what your new nose will look like, so that there are no surprises when you see yourself in the mirror.

Once you are ready, the surgery usually takes about an hour and a half and can be done in a hospital or an office setting under general or local anesthesia. All the work on your nose will be done from the inside, so you will not have any visible stitches or scarring. Your nose will be packed inside and a splint probably placed on the outside. The packing is usually removed after three or four days, but the splint will remain on from two to six days, or longer, depending on what was done.

You can expect to be in some discomfort for several days. Your doctor will prescribe appropriate painkillers. He may also instruct you to keep your head elevated and not to bend over for a while. You can also expect your new nose to be swollen for a while. It is important that you not be discouraged by what you see, because it may not represent what your nose will look like when it is completely healed. Sometimes the final contours will not appear for six months, though no one will be aware that you are still swollen.

CHIN AUGMENTATION OR MENTOPLASTY

A receding chin can give an otherwise good face a weak line. If the jaw is fundamentally normal, the receding chin is easily corrected with an implant, usually a silastic (siliconelike) bag. A pocket is made under the chin, and

QUESTIONS TO ASK YOUR DOCTOR ABOUT RHINOPLASTY

What kind of anesthesia will you use?

Where will the operation be done, in the office or in the hospital?

How long will I be hospitalized if it is done in the hospital?

What are your fees?

What will hospitalization cover?

What will my new nose look like?

How long will the packing stay in?

How long will the splint stay on?

When will I be able to wash my hair?

When can I have my hair colored?

When will I be able to wear makeup?

When can I go back to work or resume normal social activities?

What complications can I expect?

the implant is inserted. Once healed, the small scar is barely noticeable.

The operation can be done in a hospital or office setting under general or local anesthesia. It usually takes about three quarters of an hour. Chin augmentation is most often combined with another plastic-surgery procedure and choice of anesthesia and location is very often based on the total procedure.

BREAST ENLARGEMENT

Because midlife is a time of renewal, many women decide to fix things that have bothered them for years—
from a long or crooked nose to small breasts. You may
suddenly decide, "I've lived with this long enough and
now I'm going to have something done." Many surgeons
say that young women in their early twenties and
women forty and thereabouts are the ones who most
often ask for breast augmentation.

Breast augmentation is done in a hospital or in an in-
office clinic setting under local or general anesthesia. A
prosthesis is inserted *underneath* your natural breast tissue, so that your natural breast is on top of the implant.
This gives a more natural-feeling breast and, most important, leaves breast tissue free to be examined for
lumps or thickenings. The actual implant is in a sealed
"package" and contains either a saline solution or a silicone gel. The silicone in a breast implant is not to be
confused with the silicone injections of previous years
that were so dangerous. The silicone here is sealed in a
capsule, so that it cannot escape or move around.
Whether you receive a silicone prosthesis or a saline-
filled one depends on your doctor's preference and your
particular needs; this is something to discuss thoroughly
with your surgeon.

Here, too, your expectations should be realistic. You
can expect to increase the size of your breast by a cup
size, but you cannot expect to go from an "A" cup to a
"C" or "D." Discuss your expectations with your doctor.

The greatest fear in this kind of surgery is whether a
breast implant will make you any more susceptible to
breast cancer. At this time, there is no evidence that it

QUESTIONS TO ASK YOUR DOCTOR ABOUT BREAST AUGMENTATION

What kind of anesthesia will you use?

Where will the operation be done, in the office or in a hospital?

How long will I be hospitalized if it is done in the hospital?

What are your fees?

What will hospitalization cover?

What kind of implant will you use?

What kind of incision will you make?

How much larger will my breasts become?

What precautions will I have to take after surgery?

What complications should I expect and what can be done about them?

When can I resume normal activities?

---

will, and most doctors talk reassuringly on the subject. It is important to remember, however, that cancer develops over a long period of time. Breast implants, at least in large numbers, are a fairly recent phenomenon, and there is no sure way of knowing today that breast implants will not make you more susceptible to cancer fifteen or twenty years from now. Doctors do not think they will, but the question has not been answered definitively.

The other big question with this kind of surgery, especially for an older woman who is not concerned about nursing, is whether it will make your breasts less sensitive. (Nursing after breast augmentation is usually possible, but should be discussed with your doctor.) The answer is that breast augmentation will not permanently make your breasts less sensitive. Some nipple sensation will probably be lost temporarily, but will usually return. Scarring is minimal and not noticeable after a few months. The only major complication is the tendency to develop hard scar tissue. If you do develop such tissue, your surgeon can usually correct the problem, generally without further surgery, but it is a complication that occurs fairly often. Statistics vary and are not terribly reliable here. The best thing to do is to discuss how often your surgeon has experienced this complication and what he or she does about it when it occurs.

BREAST-REDUCTION SURGERY

Because of the tendency to gain weight as we age and for the breasts to become larger and droopier, breast-reduction surgery is a common midlife procedure. It is more complicated than breast augmentation and the recovery period is longer. The procedure is usually done in a hospital under general anesthesia and surgery takes three to four hours to complete. Mild to moderate discomfort is expected afterward.

There are many approaches to this operation and you should discuss which would be best in your particular case. Your surgeon will probably suggest that you lose weight before surgery if you are too heavy and recommend that you try to keep the weight off after surgery. You can expect to stay in the hospital from three to five days.

QUESTIONS TO ASK YOUR DOCTOR ABOUT BREAST-REDUCTION SURGERY

What kind of anesthesia will you use?

How long will I be hospitalized?

What will your fees be?

What will hospitalization cover?

What type of surgical approach will you use?

What kind of scarring will there be?

How much reduction can I expect?

When can I resume normal activity?

What complications can I expect?

ACTION CHECKLIST FOR COSMETIC SURGERY

- Appraise your reasons for wanting surgery, to determine whether they are realistic.

- Check around for the names of several good surgeons.

- Prepare a list of questions and make consultation appointments with at least two different doctors.

- Pick the surgeon you feel most comfortable with and follow his or her advice about what is right for your particular case.

- Lose whatever weight you need to *before* surgery.

- Give yourself adequate recovery time before you return to normal activities.

- Consider either collagen or silicone, rather than surgery, for certain types of wrinkles.

NEW TECHNIQUES IN PLASTIC SURGERY

WHAT THE EXPERTS SAY

One of the big hurdles most plastic-surgery patients face is a bad case of jitters. No matter how much confidence you may have in your surgeon, you are about to undergo surgery. Someone is going to cut your face. Quite naturally, you are apprehensive about the results. Most surgeons handle this with medication given shortly before the operation. Medication does the trick, but adds to the recovery time. If you are having surgery in a hospital, premedication for anxiety simply means that you will be groggy for a longer time following the surgery. But since the trend in plastic surgery is definitely moving to in-office procedures, having the patient as alert as possible soon after the surgery is a big asset. The patient is more relaxed about going home and more able to do so without a nasty drug "hangover."

Dr. Elliot Jacobs, a young, committed, and innovative

plastic surgeon in New York City, approaches the problem of anxiety in a unique way. He hypnotizes his patients. Dr. Jacobs does not usually tell patients he is going to hypnotize them. He finds it makes them uptight, and this is counterproductive. His goal is to relax his patients as completely as possible and to reduce the drug load he has to give them during surgery. Here are Dr. Jacobs's answers to some questions about his unique use of hypnotism.

Do patients realize they are being hypnotized?

No. They simply have a sense of relaxation and calm.

How do you go about hypnotizing a patient?

Regardless of whether I am actually able to hypnotize a patient, I feel it's important to spend some time with her before surgery, to answer any last-minute questions and to relax the patient. During this time, I am able to hypnotize most patients to some degree. I start by telling them to relax, then I try to tire the eye muscles because these muscles tire easily. I might ask a patient to stare at a particular spot and as the muscles of the eyes tire, I suggest the patient close her eyes and relax. I continue to make hypnotic suggestions until I feel the patient is satisfactorily relaxed.

Are you able to hypnotize everyone?

No, not everyone; but I am able to relax everyone. Think of it as a spectrum of relaxation. Some patients fall at one end of the spectrum, others at the other, but most fall somewhere in the middle, meaning they are fairly relaxed and in anything from a mild to a deep hypnotic state.

Can you use hypnosis during the actual surgery?

Yes. I am often able to get a patient to imagine that a hand is numb, then I ask the patient to transfer the numb sensation to certain areas of her face. Many patients are able to do this so well that they go through the surgery with only an injected local anesthetic and the effects of the hypnotism.

How do you know that a patient is hypnotized sufficiently to do this?

I give the patient little tests to do to determine how deeply she is hypnotized. For example, I might ask a patient to decrease the sensitivity in her hand. I ask her to raise one finger on the hand she chooses to numb. When the hand is numb, I instruct her to lower her finger. I explain that this will take time and I leave her alone for a few minutes while she works on the task. Even if I return to find her finger still up in the air, I know she is hypnotized because she has raised the finger. During the surgery, I might ask a patient to relive a pleasant experience. I often find patients smiling while I work because they are happily reliving some pleasant memories.

I am able to hypnotize a few patients so deeply that they actually can control the size of the small blood vessels where I am working and thus they help me control bleeding. To do this, I tell the patient that it's cold or that her face feels cold. This cold feeling causes the vessels to contract and they bleed less.

Can patients use these relaxation techniques to reduce discomfort after surgery?

Yes. I try to teach them a few self-hypnosis techniques so that they can relax themselves and reduce postoperative discomfort. Most patients tell me it works very well and they have little or no pain or discomfort.

Why don't more doctors use this technique if it works so well?

Since I don't have a hospital or operating-room schedule to restrict me, I am more able to spend the appropriate amount of time with each patient to ensure the best surgical results. Many doctors feel that they don't have the time to work with patients. I find, especially since I work in my office, that the time spent relaxing my patients is well worthwhile. They come out of operations feeling better, they are happier, and they have a much more positive attitude about the entire procedure.

LOOKING BETTER WITHOUT SURGERY

As you have discovered, cosmetic surgery is not a wrinkle eraser; yet wrinkles are often the most troublesome signs of early aging. Thanks to some new products, wrinkles can be erased easily and safely. Very recently, a California company put a new *collagen product* on the market called Zyderm. Zyderm is a form of purified cow's collagen. Cow collagen is enough like human collagen to make it successful for human use. Unlike collagen applied to the skin, this collagen is injected into a deeper layer of the skin, where it plumps up and smooths out wrinkles. Collagen injections can be used to smooth out forehead lines, crow's-feet, lines around and over the mouth. It can also be used to fill in depressions, especially those left by acne.

Shortly after collagen is injected into your skin, it actually becomes part of your skin's structure. Its makers claim that if skin injected with collagen is analyzed under a microscope, it is almost impossible to tell injected collagen from your own natural collagen. *Silicone,* another substance often injected to smooth out wrinkles, is not incorporated with your collagen.

Collagen injections have revolutionized the treatment of wrinkles. The injections are relatively inexpensive and can be done by either a dermatologist or a cosmetic surgeon in his office. The procedure is slightly uncomfortable, but not really painful. Several injections may be needed to correct a wrinkle because the collagen is mixed with a saline solution. The saline solution is absorbed by your body, causing the wrinkle to depress slightly after the original injection. Usually two to three treatments are necessary for a successful correction. If you have a lot of wrinkles, say two or three long lines in your forehead, you may have to return several times for total correction. One line at a time will usually be worked on.

ALLERGY PROBLEMS

As good as collagen seems to be, it is not without drawbacks. Some percentage of the population is allergic to it. Figures vary, depending on whom you talk to, but as much as 5 percent, or more, of the people who are tested are allergic to collagen. If you decide to have collagen treatments, your doctor will give you a *test injection,* usually on the underside of your forearm, a month before the actual treatment is scheduled to begin. You are instructed to watch the injection site for any signs of redness, swelling, or itching. The actual percentage of people allergic to collagen is difficult to determine because a certain number of the people who experience an allergic reaction do not report problems with the test, but actually turn out to be allergic to the treatment.

It is absolutely imperative that you be given a test injection before treatment. If your doctor wants to skip this precaution, find another doctor. If you turn out to be allergic, you will experience redness and swelling at the treatment site. The symptoms may persist for anywhere from a few days to several months. The makers of collagen say that, in all cases, the allergic symptoms have disappeared and have not interfered with the effects of the treatment. Still, if you are allergic, the symptoms can be troubling; and it is not advisable to proceed with treatment if any suspicion of allergy exists.

HOW LONG DO THE RESULTS LAST?

Results last longer on some people than on others and longer in some facial areas than others. In general, you can expect to lose about 10 percent of the correction a year. Patients often want to have additional injections anywhere from eighteen months to two years after initial injections. You can, of course, have as many injections over the course of time as you need to keep the treatment site smoothed out. In part, it depends on how much you "wrinkle" the treated area. If you have had injections to correct frown lines and you continue frowning a great deal, you are going to have to have the lines treated again relatively soon. In most cases, it is impossible, or at least very difficult, to stop the activity that caused the wrinkles in the first place, so you can usually count on having a series of treatments spaced out over the years if you want to keep the wrinkles smoothed out.

HOW SAFE IS COLLAGEN?

At the present time, it would seem that collagen is very safe. Studies show that the injected collagen actually becomes part of your skin's structure over time. Collagen injections, however, have been around only a short time. Extensive testing of collagen has been done, but the substance has been widely available for only a comparatively short time. No one knows what the long-term results will be. Twenty years after treatment, problems could develop. Doctors do not believe they will, but it is impossible to say absolutely that they will not at this time. The one thing physicians can say with assurance is that collagen, once injected, stays put. Unlike silicone, it does not shift or drift, causing unexpected and unwanted bumps and bulges in other parts of the face. In the early years of silicone injections, this was a great problem and caused many women considerable anguish. Collagen does not present such problems.

SILICONE: SHOULD YOU OR SHOULDN'T YOU?

Unlike collagen injections, silicone injections used to correct wrinkles and depressions have been around for years. The FDA has approved collagen (specifically, Zyderm), but it has not approved silicone—nor is it likely to. Unfortunately, silicone has become something of a political football and the prospects of it ever being approved are dim. Still, it is possible to obtain silicone injections from reputable physicians. Some doctors are taking part in a national testing program (one that has been going on for years) prior to possible approval by the FDA. The number of physicians involved in this testing program is small, and even though silicone has not been approved by the FDA many more doctors than those in the testing program are using silicone. These doctors usually purify their own silicone for injection. The early problems with silicone resulted, in large part, from using impure silicone. The material often shifted from the injection site, or the injection site became infected. The worst horror stories centered on silicone injected in massive amounts into the breasts to increase their size. This is *never* done now. The silicone used in breast augmentation is encased in a capsule so that it can't shift or cause problems.

It is possible that your dermatologist or plastic surgeon uses both silicone (purified before use) and collagen for injection. If so, how do you choose between the two? If you turn out to be allergic to collagen, you can either use the silicone or forget about this method of wrinkle-smoothing. If you are not allergic, you will probably opt for collagen, because it does have FDA approval. In making such a decision, it is wise to consider that we don't know the long-term results of collagen injections. Silicone has been around for years and if your doctor knows how to use it correctly, and if it has been adequately purified, the chances of something unpleasant happening are small. Still, silicone does occasionally shift and move within the skin and is identified as a foreign object by your body.

If you have a good doctor whom you trust, let him guide you in making a decision. In general, *small amounts* of silicone correctly injected are usually problem-free. No test is necessary before treatment, so some doctors recommend it in order to avoid the four-week waiting period. Since silicone is an inert substance, allergy is rarely a problem. Silicone injections also tend to be more lasting than collagen injections, though silicone does not last forever either. You will need several injections over the course of time to keep a wrinkle smoothed out.

C H A P T E R 8

Y O U R S M I L E
C A N M A K E
A B I G
D I F F E R E N C E

When you evaluate your looks, do it while you are smiling. A smile can light up any face, making it warm and inviting. If your smile fails to make you happy, there is a lot you can do about it now. If, for example, you were not fitted with braces as a child although your teeth are crooked or crowded, you do not have to live the second half of your life afraid to smile. New "invisible" braces are not nearly as noticeable as the old wire ones, and often a straightening job can be done within a year. Check with a good orthodontist to see what he or she recommends for your problems.

The newest and most drastic smile brightener is cosmetic bonding. Very often bonding can do in a couple of hours what braces would take years, or caps months, to accomplish. If your bite is not off and your problem is not extreme, you are a good candidate for bonding. Bonding can repair broken or cracked teeth, stained teeth, and, to some extent, crooked teeth. Very often, a tooth can be bonded rather than capped. The bonding material, called a "composite," is made of a combination of acrylic and glass in a paste form. Your dentist "sculpts" the paste onto your teeth and hardens it with a beam of ultraviolet light. The bonding is strong and long-lasting, and when a tooth is bonded, there is no need to file away a good tooth as you must when capping. Costs for bonding are usually considerably less than for capping. The biggest pleasure is that four to six teeth can be bonded in a single visit.

HOW TO FIND A DENTIST TO BOND YOUR TEETH

Not all dentists bond teeth. The procedure is so new that, especially in nonurban areas, your local dentist may not be familiar with it or, more important, skilled at it. Ask your local dental society to give you the names of several dentists in your area, or write to the American Society for Dental Aesthetics, 635 Madison Avenue, New York, N.Y. 10022.

Since bonding is permanent, be certain you pick the right dentist. Ask the dentist you select for before-and-after pictures of former patients you can see, or if possible, the names of a few patients he or she has worked on so you can see what kind of work the dentist does. Bonding is sculpting, and not everyone is equally adept. You want to know that the dentist you choose has a good aesthetic sense as well as technical skills.

WHAT THE EXPERTS SAY

Dr. Irwin Smigel, a New York City dentist, helped develop the original bonding process and now gives lectures on bonding all over the world. He is president of the American Society for Dental Aesthetics and author of *Dental Health, Dental Beauty.* Dr. Smigel is not just a wonderful dentist; he is an artist. His patients, many of them celebrities, come from all over the country to have bonding done, and when you see the results, you understand why. He works with great intensity, thoroughly absorbed in what he is doing. When he finishes, he is as pleased as his patients are with the transformations he effects. Dr. Smigel knows more about cosmetic dentistry than perhaps any dentist in the country today. Here is what he has to say about bonding.

What is the difference between bonding and veneer?

A veneer is a preformed tooth covering made of a material very similar to bonding material. Veneer is more limited than bonding because you have only the available forms to work with; you can't sculpt it. A veneer also presents more problems in adhering to teeth. The adhesive substance that holds the veneer on must adhere to the tooth and to the veneer. Bonding goes directly on the tooth so that there is only one point of adhesion, not two.

When is veneer better than bonding?

If a dentist is not adept at sculpting the bonding material, he may achieve better results with veneer. Since a veneer is pre-formed, results are predictable.

How long does either process last?

On an average, bonding or veneer lasts from five to eight years, though it often lasts much longer. When repairs need to be made, they are usually less involved and less costly than the original work. The average cap lasts from five to fifteen years.

How can bonding help as you get older?

In addition to covering the nicks, chips, and stains that are inevitable over a period of years, bonding can do one other very important thing. As we age, our teeth wear down. It's a gradual process that we don't notice from day to day, but, eventually, there is a certain appearance that's associated with age and occurs because teeth wear down. Bonding can lengthen the teeth just enough to change your expression dramatically. Whenever a good dentist bonds the teeth of an older person, he automatically lengthens the teeth just a whisper. In some cases, the teeth that lie under the "smile lines" can also be built up a bit to soften these lines.

How do you care for bonded teeth?

You shouldn't do anything with bonded teeth that you wouldn't do with unbonded teeth. Eating ice, biting on hard objects such as bones can harm any teeth and are not recommended for bonded teeth either. Apples, corn on the cob, and the like are not problems for bonded teeth, however. Because you do have a foreign body attached to your teeth, proper cleaning is important. A good toothpaste {Dr. Smigel has developed a new one, called SuperSmile, which will be available soon} is essential, and teeth should be flossed daily. Unlike capping, bonding rarely irritates gums. A cap must fit up under the gumline; bonding stops just short of the gum, so irritation is seldom a problem. Heavy smokers will experience some staining on bonded and unbonded teeth, so they must take special care; their teeth should be professionally cleaned regularly.

What can we expect of bonding in the future?

In addition to the ability to correct chips, breaks, stains, and crooked teeth, exciting new developments involving bonding are taking place. A new kind of bridge called a "Maryland" bridge has recently been developed. When a tooth is missing, a conventional bridge is used to fill the gap. Most of the time, some goldwork shows. Using bonding techniques, we are now able to fix many gaps invisibly. The metalwork is bonded to the inside of the teeth where it won't show.

CHAPTER 9

EATING — A NEW OUTLOOK; DIET, YES, DIETING, NO!

One of the reasons the word *diet* makes most of us cringe is that it is associated with deprivation. You must deprive yourself to lose weight. You can't have your cake and a bikini-worthy body, too. But weight loss is only a small part of the diet picture. There is a bigger picture, and that is what you should examine now. A diet is simply the sum total of everything you eat—no more, no less. Either you have a good diet or you have a bad one, so start thinking about a good diet now. If you learn to eat healthfully, you won't need the deprivation kind of dieting anymore. While you are learning how to eat healthfully, however, you may need to lose some weight to get down to an ideal weight you can maintain.

No one can kid you into thinking that losing weight will be easy or that you won't have to deprive yourself of some things you like while you are losing weight. Anyone who tells you that he or she has an easy way of losing weight is fooling you. Many different kinds of diets work, temporarily, and some could be considered "easy" if you feel that eating nothing but grapefruit or drinking three liquid meals a day is easy. The trouble with any of these weight-loss plans is that they won't help you keep the weight off.

To keep weight off, you must first have a *realistic idea of what you should weigh.* That is, surprisingly, the biggest hang-up for many midlife women. They are unhappy with their weight and their bodies because they compare themselves to models or even to themselves at age twenty-five.

Though many diet and nutrition experts say you should weigh for the rest of your life what you weighed in your twenties, for most of us this is an unreal expectation that adds unnecessary stress to midlife. As you grow older, you probably will put on some weight and you will probably have to adjust to this. But—and this is a big but—the amount of weight you allow yourself to gain should be small—say, five to seven pounds above your ideal weight in your twenties. You may not put this weight on until you are well past forty. Most women put on weight after menopause. Your hormone balance and your metabolism change at this point and, unless you are going to deprive yourself unrealistically for the rest of your life, you need to adjust to becoming a bit heavier. This is *not* an excuse for getting fat. If you were at your ideal weight through your twenties and thirties, gaining five pounds or so will not spoil your figure now.

In fact, as we age, most of us look better a few pounds heavier. Being too thin can make you look gaunt. The trick is to find *your new ideal weight* and to stay at that weight. To do this, you are going to have to eat somewhat less than you may be used to, and, most important, you are going to have to *increase your activity.* This is more important than what you eat. Activity not only burns up excess calories much more efficiently than constant dieting, it is necessary for good health and continued flexibility. If you think that increased activity equals exercise, you are right. But remember, not all exercise has to be the down-on-the-floor grunt-and-groan type. There are many kinds of exercise you can build into your life, but unless you are an athletic-oriented person, you may always feel that exercise of any kind is a pain in the neck. So be it. Most of us probably feel that way, but if you are going to maintain a healthy, trim body, you will need to make some concessions to exercise. Exercise is built into the weight-loss plan that follows, but it is the easiest kind to do and it does burn up calories *and* keeps you aerobically and physically fit. You will find that if you continue the exercise plan outlined here after you have lost the weight you want, you will be able to consume more calories without putting any weight back on. Being able to eat a little more, rather than having to continue dieting, is a very good reason to exercise regularly.

HOW MUCH SHOULD YOU WEIGH?

The right answer to this question can make a big difference in your life over the next decades. It can mean the difference between being constantly unhappy and being at peace with yourself. Be realistic. If you expect to weigh what you did at twenty when you are forty-five, you are probably asking too much. In fact, your expectations at twenty may have been unrealistic.

For years, the Metropolitan Insurance Companies have told us all what we should weigh. Their tables represented ideal weights for a healthy, long life. The suggested weights had nothing to do with model-perfect figures; they reflected health. Women often were not satisfied when their weight matched the tables because they wanted to look like the superthin models in magazines. Today even models weigh more than in the past. A heavier, more athletic body is considered ideal, and that is good news. In addition, Metropolitan Life has revised its weight tables upward a bit because it found that good health could still be maintained at a slightly heavier weight. Find your height and bone structure on the chart on page 183 and see what your weight range should be. Your goal, if you are overweight, should be to come within this range, probably at the low end, or maybe slightly below the low end if you have a very small frame. The higher figures are usually too high to satisfy most women, though these higher weights are still considered healthy.

HOW TO DETERMINE YOUR BODY FRAME BY ELBOW BREADTH

To make a simple approximation of your frame size:

Extend your arm in front of you and bend the forearm upward at a 90-degree angle. Keep the fingers straight and turn the inside of your wrist away from the body. Place the thumb and index finger of your other hand on the two prominent bones on *either side* of your elbow. Measure the space between your fingers against a ruler or a tape measure. Compare the measurements on the following tables.

These tables list the elbow measurements for medium-framed women of various heights. Measurements lower than those listed indicate you have a small frame, and higher measurements indicate a large frame.

Height in 1″ heels	Elbow Breadth
4′10″–4′11″	2¼″–2½″
5′0″–5′3″	2¼″–2½″
5′4″–5′7″	2⅜″–2⅝″
5′8″–5′11″	2⅜″–2⅝″
6′0″	2½″–2¾″

WHY IS IT HARDER TO CONTROL YOUR WEIGHT NOW?

If you find that you are heavier now than you would like to be, you are not alone. There are both physiological and social reasons behind midlife weight gain. First of all, you need to realize that your basal metabolism (the rate at which your body burns calories) slows down about 3 percent from ages twenty-two to thirty-five. After this, it decreases more rapidly with each passing decade. This means that as you age, *you need fewer calories to maintain your weight*. Combine this with the fact that you are probably more sedentary now than you were ten

METROPOLITAN
HEIGHT AND WEIGHT TABLE FOR
WOMEN

Height: Feet	Inches	Small Frame	Medium Frame	Large Frame
4	10	102–111	109–121	118–131
4	11	103–113	111–123	120–134
5	0	104–115	113–126	122–137
5	1	106–118	115–129	125–140
5	2	108–121	118–132	128–143
5	3	111–124	121–135	131–147
5	4	114–127	124–138	134–151
5	5	117–130	127–141	137–155
5	6	120–133	130–144	140–159
5	7	123–136	133–147	143–163
5	8	126–139	136–150	146–167
5	9	129–142	139–153	149–170
5	10	132–145	142–156	152–173
5	11	135–148	145–159	155–176
6	0	138–151	148–162	158–179

Weights at Ages 25–59.
Based on Lowest Mortality. Weight in Pounds According to Frame (in indoor clothing weighing 3 lbs., shoes with 1″ heels).
Reprinted with permission of the Metropolitan Insurance Companies

years ago, and consider that you probably also have more social occasions to eat well. Most of us do a major part of our socializing over a good meal. As we get older, more of this eating tends to be done in restaurants, where we usually exercise less control over what we eat and where the temptations to eat are greater. Add all this up, and you can see why it is so easy to put on pounds now. Unless you want to be on a constant diet, not a healthy or realistic situation, the only way you can control your weight is to increase your activity level. You can do this while still eating *relatively* normally.

WHY SHOULD YOU EAT?

Many women have mistaken ideas about the food they eat. Many of us have grown up with the idea that bread and starches are the first things that should go when we are on a diet. In the past few years, we have learned a great deal about what our bodies need to stay healthy and trim. Carbohydrates, we have learned, should not be the first thing we eliminate. In fact, 58 percent of your daily intake should be composed of complex carbohydrates (fresh fruits and vegetables and whole grains). A diet high in protein—the old high-protein reducing-diet idea—is no longer considered healthy. Most Americans eat far too much protein. Forty-four grams a day, about the amount in two glasses of milk plus a three-ounce individual can of tuna, is now considered adequate. One of the main reasons a high-protein diet is not desirable is that so many popular protein foods contain as many or more fat calories as they do protein. For example, we used to think that a steak was good diet food, but even a lean steak contains a lot of fat. A five-ounce steak contains about 536 calories, compared to 200 calories for the same amount of spaghetti with meat sauce. If you are going to eat for health, it is important that you understand that every gram of fat you eat has more than twice the number of calories as a gram of carbohydrate or protein. One gram of fat contains nine calories, and a gram of carbohydrate—or a gram of protein—contains only four calories.

Eating a high-protein diet also does not provide your body with the valuable vitamins and minerals and fiber that carbohydrates provide. Most of us could cut down the amount of protein we eat by half and still consume an adequate amount. Likewise, we could double the amount of carbohydrates we eat and probably still not be eating as much as nutrition experts recommend today.

Although counting calories is a boring way to stay thin, if you don't know something about calories, you are going to have a very difficult time controlling your weight. It is a good idea to *buy a good calorie-counting book* and leaf through it to gain an idea of where the big calorie loads are coming from. You will discover that it is not the pasta that is fattening; it is the oil, butter, or cheese you add to it. It is not the baked potato that is high in calories; it is the sour cream or the pats of butter you eat with it. You also will learn that your favorite "innocent" salad may contain a lot more calories than you thought if it's loaded with oily dressing. You will also understand why everyone tells you to eat chicken and fish as often as you can while skipping fat-laden steaks, chops, and roasts. You will see, too, why not eating dessert makes such good sense. Desserts are calorie disasters because most are loaded with butter, eggs, or cream that deliver far more calories than the sugar most people believe to be the worst culprit.

EATING FOR MIDLIFE

There are many formulas that tell you how to count calories for weight maintenance. Some are quite complicated and involve multiplying your weight by a certain number of calories. These formulas probably work, but they make you count calories constantly, and most of us do not have the discipline for this. It is far better to acquaint yourself with the highly caloric foods and try to avoid them as much as possible, and to learn what portion size and food varieties you can eat and still maintain a good weight. The most important thing is to balance eating with activity on a weekly basis. If you have a fairly sedentary week, compensate by cutting back calories for a few days. You will find it easiest and most effective to think of eating and exercising in weekly units. Weighing yourself every day is a drag and discouraging. Your weight can fluctuate several pounds a day because of water buildup. This can make you panic and think you've gained when, in fact, you have not. Weighing yourself once a week will help you keep your weight in check; when you find you are moving too far up on the scale, cut back calories and increase your exercise.

Eating for midlife is not just a matter of calories, however. One of the most important changes at this time of your life involves bone density. One woman out of four is going to suffer from *osteoporosis*, a degenerative bone disorder that reduces bone mass, making bones brittle and extremely prone to breakage. Osteoporosis causes many elderly women to break their hips, arms, ankles, and legs more readily than their male counterparts. Experts used to think that calcium loss did not start until midlife; new studies show this is not true. Many young women in their twenties are already losing bone, but the loss intensifies after menopause. A woman can lose 10 to 15 percent of her bone mass in each of the first few years after menopause. Victims are unaware of the loss, usually well into old age, by which time the loss has become so acute that the simplest accident causes bones to break. Doctors now know that many women who "fall" and break their hips do not fall at all. The fragile hip bone, after losing so much of its mass, simply fractures spontaneously, and it is the fracture that causes the fall.

Grim as this may sound, there is something you can do about it. If you have a family history of osteoporosis, you should have a serious talk with your doctor about *estrogen-replacement therapy*. Research indicates that this therapy does much to prevent the bone loss that occurs after menopause. If your doctor is against such therapy, talk to at least one other doctor. Attitudes are changing about estrogen therapy, and osteoporosis is so disabling that it is worthwhile to be certain you have accurately appraised the pros and cons in your particular case. A second doctor may feel it is worthwhile and safe for you to take estrogen to prevent bone problems.

Even if you can't or don't want to take estrogen, you can still do a great deal to help prevent osteoporosis. Doctors believe women should be getting from 1,200 to 1,400 milligrams of calcium a day (the amount in four glasses of milk). The average woman, however, usually only takes in three to five hundred milligrams a day. Clearly, you need to increase your intake dramatically if you are not to come up short. Good natural sources of calcium, besides dairy products, are green leafy vegetables, nuts, raisins, dates, and fish that contain tiny bones like sardines and canned salmon. Tofu, a bean curd used in Oriental cooking, is an excellent source. Even with a fairly healthy diet, the chances are that you still are not going to get an adequate amount of calcium. A calcium supplement, then, is the only way to get it. You should take supplemental calcium with vitamin D, because adequate amounts of this vitamin are essential for absorbing calcium. Since you will undoubtedly be cutting down on total calories during midlife, it makes good sense to take a daily multivitamin (one that supplies no more than 100 percent of the recommended daily allowance of vitamins and minerals) with a calcium supplement. If you get into the habit of taking both just before breakfast and make it part of your daily routine, you will never forget to take your vitamins. Taking calcium supplements does not guarantee that you will never get osteoporosis, but it certainly helps. In addition, you should also avoid excess caffeine, salt, and tobacco. All these substances reduce your body's ability to absorb calcium.

You have already read about the case for exercise in helping you control your weight. There is another very important reason why you need to exercise more at this time in your life. Exercise is vital to the formation of new bone. Researchers have found, for example, that tennis players have thicker bones in the arm they hit the ball with. One of the best exercises for allover bone formation is walking. Long, brisk walks are not only good for your heart, lungs, and figure, but also for your bones. Actually, any exercise you like—and, therefore, will do—is fine.

One additional aspect of nutrition to keep in mind at this time in your life is fiber consumption. Most Americans don't get enough fiber; as you get older, fiber is important for regularity. Eating lots of fresh fruits and vegetables and whole grains is the surest way to ingest enough fiber.

THE TEN-POUNDS-OFF REWARD DIET

Do you reward yourself with food? If you are interested in this diet, the chances are that you do. We are all taught to reward ourselves with food, from the time we are infants. When babies or children cry, they often get fed. When you were a child, you probably got rewarded for good behavior by being allowed to have your favorite food. If you cleaned your plate, you got dessert. Because this kind of reward process is so ingrained in most of us, we spend our adult lives rewarding ourselves with food. We do it when we are depressed, frustrated, angry—and we get fat. This diet is unique because it embodies the reward concept while it retrains you to think about what constitutes a reward.

This diet is called a "reward" diet because you are allowed one "reward" each day. The reward principle is central to the success of the diet, because it gives you a choice to make—and feeling you have a choice on a diet is important. It also gives you something to look forward to every day. But, most important, it trains you to rethink your idea of a reward. Anyone can think of pie with ice cream as a reward; on this diet, you will learn to lower your expectations to something less extravagant. A diet milk shake or "float" made with diet ingredients can fulfill your need to be rewarded and still not blow your diet. Even a couple of pretzels or a few potato chips can be savored as a reward when you learn to scale down your expectations of how much of a reward you can give yourself. No matter what reward you pick from those allowed on the diet, you must teach yourself to savor it, to appreciate it as much as you would a piece of cake or a slice of pie. This may seem hard at first, but you can do it. It is a lot easier than cutting out *all* rewards and never allowing yourself to have any of your favorite foods.

Before starting this or *any* diet, check with your doctor to be certain you have no health problems that would make dieting harmful. If you follow this diet carefully, you can lose ten pounds in about five weeks, or even less, depending on how much you exercise and how much you weigh at the outset. It is a nutritionally sound diet that will give you vitamins and minerals plus fiber; but, if you plan to stay on it for more than two weeks, it is a good idea to take a multivitamin daily, if you are not already taking one. You really should take a daily multivitamin on a regular basis after forty, but it is especially important whenever you diet, no matter what weight-loss plan you are following, because it is difficult to get all the nutrients you need on any reduced-calorie diet.

You do not have to count calories on this diet. Each day's intake equals approximately 1,200 calories, including your daily reward. You have options, however, so on certain days, depending on what options you pick, your calories may run just under or just over 1,200.

You will lose approximately two pounds a week. If you exercise regularly, you will lose faster. Also, the heavier you are, the faster you will lose, especially when you first start the diet. The more you weigh, the more calories it takes to maintain that weight, so if you cut down to 1,200, you will lose more weight at first than a woman who weighs less and needs fewer calories to fuel her body.

Foods on the Ten-Pounds-Off Reward Diet are tasty and flavorful. The dinners, especially, are designed to be satisfying in texture and flavor. You may be surprised to see two slices of bread on each day's diet and to discover that you can eat rice and pasta. These complex carbohydrates are not only tasty and filling, they are healthy and relatively low in calories. You must, however, be accurate about portion size and the amount of sauce or spread you use—that is where the calories pile up.

YOUR DIET SHOPPING LIST

Many of the things you will be eating will be staples you buy regularly, but the following items are necessary and may not be on your regular shopping list.

Diet margarine

Diet jelly

Diet mayonnaise

Low-fat milk

Diet cheese slices

Several kinds of diet salad dressing

Pam spray

Soy sauce, preferably light soy sauce which is salt reduced

Fresh ginger root

A large, nonstick frying pan

MEALS

The following weekly meal plan will work for you if you are the kind of dieter who needs to be told exactly what to eat. If you do not like following such a rigid plan, you can pick from the optional Alternate Meals, or eat lunch at dinnertime and vice versa. If you work, you can select the lunch menus that are easiest to obtain in a restaurant or to carry in a "brown bag." You can eat Tuesday's plan on Thursday or mix the days any way you like—with the exception of Saturday and Sunday. These two days' meals have higher calorie counts and you should eat them on weekends only (or twice a week only). You may drink as much coffee, tea, and diet soda as you wish. Use sugar substitute to sweeten beverages, and nondairy creamers. One special feature of the diet and an idea you should build into your lifelong eating plan is the heavy reliance on fish, chicken, and veal rather than on beef and pork, which contain more fat.

MONDAY

Breakfast

½ grapefruit, or a small glass grapefruit or tomato juice

¾ cup dry cereal (any unsugared variety, but vitamin- and fiber-enriched varieties are preferred) with ½ cup low-fat milk

1 slice whole-grain toast, spread lightly with diet margarine and diet jelly

Midmorning

1 small piece of fruit

Lunch

Individual-serving can of tuna (3 oz.), packed in water
1 small tomato, crudités (carrot sticks, celery, etc.)
1 slice plain whole-grain bread

Midafternoon

1 slice diet cheese

Dinner, Sautéed Chicken

1 small chicken breast, boneless and skinless, cut into
slivers or diced
Diet margarine or Pam
1 tablespoon light soy sauce
2 tablespoons chopped scallions or chives

Sauté chicken in nonstick pan with a little diet margarine or Pam and a tablespoon of soy sauce to moisten.
Add scallions or chives.

Serve with 1 cup steamed broccoli, seasoned with
lemon juice and a sprinkle of Parmesan cheese, and a
mixed green salad tossed with diet dressing.

1 reward, to be eaten anytime.

TUESDAY

Breakfast

½ grapefruit or a small glass tomato or grapefruit juice
1 soft-boiled egg

1 slice whole-grain toast, spread lightly with diet margarine and diet jelly

Midmorning
1 small piece of fruit

Lunch
¾ cup low-fat cottage cheese

½ cup mixed fruit cocktail, packed in water

1 slice whole-grain bread

Midafternoon
1 slice diet cheese

2 whole-grain crackers

Dinner, Gingered Fish
1 large fish fillet—sole, flounder, fluke, or scrod

1 tablespoon diet margarine or Pam

1 tablespoon light soy sauce

2 tablespoons chopped shallots or chives

½-inch piece of peeled fresh ginger, minced fine

Sauté fish in nonstick pan with margarine or Pam and soy sauce to moisten. Add chopped shallots or chives and ginger.

Serve with 1 cup steamed green beans, sprinkled with a teaspoon grated Parmesan cheese, and a mixed green salad tossed with diet dressing.

1 reward, to be eaten anytime.

WEDNESDAY

Breakfast

1 8-oz. container of yogurt—coffee, vanilla, lemon, lime, or plain (do *not* use any other flavors of yogurt, especially those with fruit preserves)

1 slice whole-grain toast, spread lightly with diet margarine

Midmorning

1 small piece of fruit

Lunch

4 slices fresh chicken or turkey (avoid commercial turkey or chicken roll because of their high salt content)

1 slice whole-grain bread

1 hard-cooked egg

Crudités

Midafternoon

1 slice of diet cheese

Dinner, Veal Paillard

1 large, lean veal chop, "butterflied" for Veal Paillard, or 1 medium (about 4 oz.) veal scaloppine

Diet margarine or Pam
Chopped parsley

Broil the veal, basting lightly with diet margarine, or sauté in diet margarine or Pam in a nonstick pan. Garnish with chopped parsley.

Serve with ½ cup steamed brown rice and a green salad with diet dressing.

1 reward, to be eaten whenever you like.

THURSDAY

Breakfast
Repeat Monday's breakfast.

Midmorning
1 small piece of fruit

Lunch
Cheese sandwich made with 3 slices diet cheese or 2 slices regular cheese and 1 slice whole-grain bread spread with mustard
Crudités, pickles

Midafternoon
Small box raisins

Dinner, Chicken with Ginger
1 small boneless, skinless chicken breast
1 tablespoon diet margarine
1 tablespoon light soy sauce
½-inch piece of peeled fresh ginger, minced fine
Pinch of dried, minced garlic

To prepare garlic chicken, cut chicken breast into shoestring slices and sauté in a nonstick pan in diet margarine and soy sauce. Add minced ginger and garlic.

Serve with ½ cup steamed brown rice and a green salad with diet dressing.

1 reward, eaten when desired.

FRIDAY

Breakfast
Repeat Tuesday's breakfast.

Midmorning
1 small piece of fruit

Lunch
Lean hamburger, well drained of grease, on half a roll or 1 slice whole-grain bread

½ cup fruit cocktail, packed in water

Midafternoon
1 slice diet cheese

2 whole-grain crackers

Dinner, Liver and Onions
2 medium slices (3–4 oz.) calves' liver

1 small onion, chopped

1 tablespoon diet margarine

1 teaspoon dry vermouth (optional)

Sauté the liver and the onion in diet margarine. You may add a teaspoon of dry vermouth to moisten, but let simmer for a minute to allow the alcohol—and the calories—to evaporate.

Serve with 1 cup steamed green beans, seasoned with lemon juice and your favorite herbs, and a green salad tossed with diet dressing.

1 reward, eaten when desired.

SATURDAY

Breakfast
Repeat Wednesday's breakfast.

Midmorning
1 small piece of fruit

Lunch
½ grapefruit

4 thin slices (3–4 oz.) lean roast beef on 1 slice toasted whole-grain bread spread lightly with diet mayonnaise, margarine, and/or mustard

Crudités

Dinner
Pasta Primavera

1 cup cooked pasta (any kind)

1 cup steamed vegetables (diced broccoli, green beans, asparagus, cauliflower—whatever "allowed" vegetables you like)

2 tablespoons diet margarine

1 tablespoon grated Parmesan cheese

Toss pasta and vegetables with margarine and Parmesan cheese. You can keep the dish from getting cold before it is served by tossing the margarine and cheese with the pasta and vegetables in your frying pan over low heat. Serve with a green salad and diet dressing.

1 reward, eaten when you like.

SUNDAY

Breakfast

½ grapefruit, or small glass of grapefruit, tomato, or orange juice

2 slices cinnamon toast (toast whole-grain bread, spread lightly with diet margarine, then sprinkle with sugar and cinnamon mixed together)

1 scrambled egg (made in a nonstick pan sprayed with Pam)

Midmorning

1 small piece of fruit

Lunch

1 cup canned chili (compare labels before buying, as calorie counts vary tremendously), served with saltines

½ cup fresh fruit salad

Dinner, Steak and Potato

1 small (5–6 oz.) lean steak, trimmed of fat and broiled

1 medium baked potato, with 1 tablespoon diet margarine

Green salad with diet dressing

Bedtime

Small glass of low-fat milk

1 reward, eaten when you like.

REWARDS

You may pick anything from this list to have once a day. You may not have more than two starred items in a week. Have your reward anytime you like. You might prefer the sweet rewards as dessert after dinner. The snack-type rewards might be pleasurable in the evening while you are reading or watching television. You might also prefer to set aside some private time for yourself, free of family interruptions or work worries. You could enjoy your reward during this time, making the private time and the food part of your reward system.

You can stretch your reward by combining it with some no-calorie food. For instance, if you have picked potato chips or pretzels, you might have them with a diet soda or a glass of sparkling water flavored with a fresh lime slice. If you have chosen cookies, you might have them with a cup of tea or coffee (use a nondairy-type creamer). If you have selected an alcoholic beverage for a reward, serve it in a small wineglass, to give you the feeling you are getting more.

4 oz. wine

3 oz. dry sherry

8 oz. light beer

6 potato chips

2 sugar cookies

2 chocolate-chip cookies

3 chocolate-covered graham crackers

Reward shake: In a blender, combine 1 cup low-fat milk, ½ tsp. vanilla or almond extract, 2 tsp. sugar, and ice cubes. Blend till foamy.

*½ cup ice milk

*½ cup fruit sherbet

1 cup consommé or bouillon spiked with 1 oz. sherry or port

Any fresh fruit

4 pretzels

1 cup unbuttered popcorn

*Pear Tropical: Marinate 1 sliced ripe pear in rum to cover for a few hours. Eat pear, but don't spoon up the marinade; have only what clings to pear slices. You may sweeten a little with sugar substitute if you like.

*Orange Delight: Peel, section, and seed an orange and marinate for several hours in enough orange liqueur to cover. Eat the orange and whatever marinade clings to slices. Don't spoon up excess marinade.

Cinnamon Apple: Peel and slice a medium apple; sprinkle very lightly with sugar, and generously with cinnamon.

Ice-Cream Soda: Add 1 heaping tablespoon ice milk to a glass of ice-cold diet ginger ale.

Cappuccino Float: Add 1 tablespoon ice milk to cup of hot or cold strong coffee or espresso. Sprinkle cinnamon on top.

Sailor's Tea: One cup hot tea spiked with 1 teaspoon rum and sugar substitute.

ALTERNATE MEALS

Pick any of these additional dinners to stretch and add variety to your diet menu.

Stir-Fry Chicken and Vegetables

1 chicken breast, skinless and boneless

1 tablespoon oil

¼ cup broccoli

¼ cup green beans

¼ cup asparagus or cauliflower

1 tablespoon light soy sauce

Few slices water chestnut

Over high heat in a nonstick pan coated with one tablespoon oil, sauté the broccoli, green beans, and the asparagus or cauliflower for one minute. Add chicken breast, diced or cut in shoestring slices. Add 1 tablespoon light soy sauce and a few slices of water chestnut, drained. Stir well and sauté until chicken is cooked and vegetables are crisp-tender.

Serve with ½ cup steamed rice and a green salad with diet dressing.

Fish Chowder

1 fish fillet (sole, flounder, or scrod are good choices)

1 small onion

1 tablespoon diet margarine

2 small boiled potatoes, diced

1 cup low-fat milk

fresh parsley for garnish

Chop and sauté a small onion in margarine until soft. Add diced potatoes. In another pot, heat the milk; add fish and simmer gently until the fish flakes. Add onion and potato. Garnish with fresh parsley.

Serve with 3 whole-grain crackers and a green salad with diet dressing.

Curried Tuna or Chicken Salad

1 boneless, skinless chicken breast OR 1 individual-serving can (3 oz.) tuna, packed in water

2 stalks celery, diced

1 scallion, diced

½ teaspoon curry powder

1 tablespoon diet mayonnaise

1 large, ripe tomato

Poach and dice the chicken breast; or use tuna packed in water. Add cooled chicken or the tuna to diced celery and scallion in a bowl. Add ½ teaspoon curry powder (or more or less, to taste), and mayonnaise. Combine all ingredients well and stuff into the tomato. You can substitute a handful of grapes and raisins for the celery and onion, if you prefer.

Serve the salad with one slice of whole-grain toast (remember: limit bread to two slices a day) or, if you've already eaten your allowed quantity of bread, with 3 whole-grain crackers.

ALTERNATE "ALLOWED" VEGETABLES

You can substitute any of the following vegetables for those called for in the meal plan:

Asparagus
Broccoli
Brussels sprouts
Carrots
Cauliflower
Collards
Green beans
Kale
Parsnips
Spinach
Turnip greens
Turnips
Zucchini

AEROBIC WALKING TO MELT OFF POUNDS

There is a hitch to any diet, and this one is no different. You *will* lose weight if you follow the eating plan, but you will lose faster if you exercise, too. Not only will exercise help you lose excess weight faster, it will help you keep that weight off when you resume more normal eating. The exercise most people find easiest, believe it or not, is plain old walking!

Walking is a lost art. We step into our cars to go to a shopping center a mile away. We ride in crowded buses or subways to get to work. Don't ride! Start walking and watch the pounds melt away. By walking, I don't mean a leisurely stroll down Main Street. *Aerobic walking* is what is needed to melt the weight away. You should walk at least two miles a day—four is ideal—four to five times a week to attain aerobic benefits. Walking two miles should take you about thirty minutes if you walk at a good clip. If it takes you much longer, you are not walking fast enough to get aerobic benefits. You must also *walk continuously*. No stopping and starting. If you live in a city, figure twenty city blocks equals a mile. If you work, the best way to get your walking in is to walk at lunch or walk to work, or at least part of the way. If you drive, park your car two miles from your office and walk the last two miles. You will double your benefits if you also walk the two miles to your car at night. But if you can't do this, you can take public transportation to the spot where you parked your car, or perhaps you can persuade a friend to drive you to your car. Another solution is to take public transportation, but get off the bus or train two miles before you normally would. Do the same thing coming home. However you work out the logistics, you must get in at least two miles of fast walking at one time.

If you are not a walker, two miles will seem like a long way at first, but after a week, you will be surprised how fast it goes. You will be at your destination before you know it. Walking is also a wonderful way to clear your mind or solve problems. If you have a busy work schedule or a lot of family or community responsibilities, it can be your very own time to think your own thoughts.

Walking is wonderful exercise and once you get into the groove, you will find you truly enjoy it. It is also exercise you can do for the rest of your life. You can, however, do any kind of aerobic exercise that you find pleasurable. You can bike for a half hour a day, swim laps for a half hour, jog for twenty minutes, even skip rope for twenty minutes if you like. You can vary these activities seasonally or weekly, *but you must exercise regularly.*

You can easily figure out how many calories walking burns off for you. If you are walking the ideal four miles daily, and walking that distance in an hour, multiply your weight by 2.35. If you are a 120-pound woman, that means four miles of walking burns off approximately 282 calories a day. Do this five times a week and you have burned off about 1,400 extra calories. You can see that is more calories than you eat in one day of dieting! This means you will lose weight much faster than by dieting alone.

HOW TO KEEP THE WEIGHT OFF

Once you have lost the weight you wanted to, don't do what so many people do—start eating just as you did before. If you were fat before, that kind of eating is going to make you fat again. The most sensible thing to do is slowly begin to add additional calories to your diet and see what happens to your weight. If you don't gain, you can handle that amount of calories. If you start gaining, you must cut back a bit.

If you have started to retrain yourself to lower-calorie food rewards, in place of the higher-calorie ones, you are already off to a good start. To reinforce this behavior, continue to use the reward foods in the Ten-Pounds-Off Reward Diet for several months after you have actually stopped dieting. Whenever you feel like treating yourself to a high-calorie reward, substitute your favorite reward from the diet's allowed reward list. Continue to limit the amount of fat-laden red meat you eat. Don't have marbled steaks, roasts, or chops unless it is unavoidable—for example, if you are at someone else's home for a meal. If you have a longing for red meat, or you cook for a family that can't live without it, trim as much of the fat from your portion as possible. Remember that lean pork—pigs are being bred to produce leaner meat—is often a better choice than marbled beef. Experiment with different recipes for fish and chicken. Both are low-calorie, low in fat, and can be prepared in dozens of different ways. Veal is always a good choice, but it is expensive. Try the least-expensive cuts or scaloppine (not cheap, but you don't need much) or some roasts.

If you still feel your calorie-counting expertise is lacking, pull out your calorie book and bone up. Becoming totally familiar with the calorie pitfalls is absolutely necessary if you are to control your weight. Once you are familiar with the caloric and nutritional values of common foods, you are much more likely to eat a healthy diet.

Still, the most important weight controller is exercise. If you are not committed to some form now, you are missing your best shot at weight control. So many women have discovered its value—why shouldn't you be one of them? Jill, a forty-two-year-old business-woman, says, "I hated the idea that I had to exercise to stay in shape, but I also hated the way I was starting to look. Reluctantly, I bought myself a pair of running shoes and started walking to work every day. Now I treasure my morning and evening walk. I mull over the day's problems or just enjoy the feeling the exercise gives me. It's actually become one of the best parts of my day." Helen, a fifty-year-old housewife, has a different attitude. "I hate exercising. I always have, I always will, but I refuse to get out of shape and I see that as soon as I give up my daily run in the park, the pounds start sliding on. You can't always like everything in your life; there are just some things you have to do, that's all."

THE FIVE-POUND SOLUTION

One of the reasons it can be so difficult to lose weight and keep it off is that you let the problem become acute before you do anything about it. The five-pound solution keeps you from doing this. After you have reached your ideal weight, weigh yourself once a week. Don't allow yourself to gain more than five pounds. As soon as you see the scale creeping toward that five-pound mark, go back on the Reward Diet until you are back at your ideal weight. This way you will never have a large chunk of weight to lose. Try going on the Reward Diet two weeks before you go away on vacation, too, so that you won't have to lose weight *after* you come back. Your motivation is much greater when you have a vacation to look forward to.

ACTION CHECKLIST FOR GOOD NUTRITION AND THE RIGHT WEIGHT

- Decide what your ideal weight should be.

- Go on the Ten-Pounds-Off Reward Diet if you are over your ideal weight.

- Increase your activity level to help control weight.

- Become familiar with calorie counts of common foods and with food traps.

- Increase your consumption of complex carbohydrates and lower your consumption of high-fat protein foods.

- Take a multivitamin and a calcium supplement daily.

- Adopt the Five-Pound Solution as a lifelong weight-control measure.

WHAT THE EXPERTS SAY

Jane Kirby makes nutrition a feminist issue. Her knowledge of food and nutrition as it relates to women is extensive, and she is passionate about educating women about it. A registered dietitian who worked at the prestigious Massachusetts General Hospital, Ms. Kirby also worked for the *Ladies' Home Journal* and *Good Housekeeping* and is currently the innovative food and nutrition editor of *Glamour* magazine. Here is what she has to say about eating at midlife.

What basic eating changes should you make at midlife?

Most young women get by nicely on a diet of about 2,000 calories a day. Sometime between forty and fifty, depending on your body, you should reduce your calories to about 1,800.

Is it difficult to get all the nutrients you need with this number of calories?

Yes it is, especially if you're not nutritionally savvy. For this reason, it's wise to take a multivitamin pill daily. It's also important to remember to take your pill while there is food in your stomach. A vitamin on an empty stomach—so many people take them before bed or early in the morning—doesn't do much good. You need food in your stomach for the vitamin to work most effectively.

Does your need for particular nutrients change at midlife?

Yes. After menopause, you need less iron than you did previously, but it's still difficult to get enough following the diets most of us eat. A multivitamin plus iron is still a good idea. Remember to consume vitamin-C–rich foods—citrus fruits and tomatoes are good C sources—when you take iron. Vitamin C enhances the absorption of iron. New research indicates that vitamin E is useful in coping with certain menopausal symptoms, mainly hot flashes. Nuts, dark-green leafy vegetables, especially broccoli, are good sources. You may want to discuss taking a vitamin E supplement with your doctor.

You also need more calcium as you get older. It's a good idea for most older women to take a calcium supplement and be certain that they are getting enough vitamin D. This vitamin is necessary for the absorption of calcium. Dairy products are good sources of vitamin D and calcium. If you take a calcium supplement, don't be put off by the size of the pills and the number you need to take to meet the RDA. Because of its structure, it's impossible to get calcium into a small pill. This means you may be taking a half dozen hefty pills a day. You can take them a few at a time throughout the day to avoid taking them all at once. Look for calcium lactate or calcium carbonate, not dolomite. Dolomite, a common calcium supplement, has been found to contain harmful amounts of arsenic and lead.

What other changes in eating should you make at midlife?

Women at midlife, and well before, should reduce the amount of fat in their diets, both saturated and unsaturated fat. New research seems to link incidence of breast cancer with high-fat diets. In countries where the national diet is low in fat—such as Japan—breast cancer is less common.

Why is it important to eat well at midlife?

It is very important to follow good nutritional habits at any age, but between forty and fifty, it is especially important. During our twenties and thirties, our systems are often nutritionally depleted because of our hectic schedules and because of childbearing. We have the decade between forty and fifty to get into good nutritional shape so that we are as fit and healthy as possible when we go through the menopause. It is important to be nutritionally healthy at this time of physical and emotional stress.

How many calories should you consume when you diet during this period of your life?

Most researchers feel that a reducing diet of around 1,200 calories a day works best. Reducing calories more makes it tough to get proper nutrition; even at 1,200 calories, you must choose your foods very carefully. After forty, or certainly around fifty, you probably need to reduce calories to about 1,000 to lose weight, depending on your body size. Your metabolism has slowed down and you're likely to be more sedentary, so a 1,000-calorie-a-day diet is about the level for most women to lose weight. At this calorie level, however, a multivitamin is necessary. Also, do not stay on a diet this low in calories for too long.

C H A P T E R   10

E X E R C I S E   H I T S
T H E   S P O T

If you have lumps, bumps, and bulges—and it is perfectly possible to have them, even if you are at your ideal weight—the only way to make them disappear is to start a program of good spot exercises. Spot exercises are meant to tone and firm a particular area such as upper thighs, stomach, and so forth. Doing the exercises may not be your favorite pastime, but the results justify the effort.

Before you start, be realistic about your expectations. If you are generally overweight, don't expect a few exercises to be a cure-all. Your body will not slim and trim down without diet and aerobic exercise combined. But if you have achieved your ideal weight or are working toward it, doing these spot exercises will make you happier with the shape of your body. They can firm up sagging thigh muscles, pull in a bulgy tummy, and whittle away at a thickened waist.

To do the exercises, you will need to lie on the floor, so either buy yourself an exercise mat or lie on a thick rug or carpet; exercising on too hard a surface can be damaging to your back. When you are on your back, always be sure to keep your entire spine pressed against the floor. Do not let the small of your back curve up. Breathe deeply as you exercise and keep your movements slow and rhythmical, rather than quick and jerky. You should run through this series of exercises three or four times a week. Here goes!

THIGH AND BUTTOCKS FIRMERS

This area is probably the one that causes more problems for women than any other. A sagging fanny or that little giveaway spread on your thigh, just at the bathing-suit line, can be a real figure spoiler. These exercises work both areas, so you get two for one!

THIGHS AND BUTTOCKS FIRMER

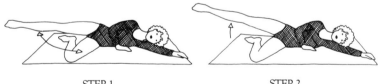

STEP 1   STEP 2

1. Lie on your left side, stretched out on the floor with your left arm stretched over your head. Your right arm should be bent, with the palm down on the floor. Now bend your knees so that your legs form a right angle to your body. Straighten and bend your right leg, keeping it at hip level. Repeat 15 times. Do not allow leg to touch floor at any time.

2. Lie as above, but this time raise and lower your right leg slowly, again not letting right leg touch floor when you lower it. Keep your toe pointed down toward the floor. Repeat 15 times.

3. Repeat both exercises on opposite side.

STOMACH FIRMERS

Because of childbirth and the aging process, many women end up at forty with weak stomach muscles, causing their stomachs to bulge unattractively. These exercises are terrific for firming and tightening those weak muscles.

STOMACH FIRMER

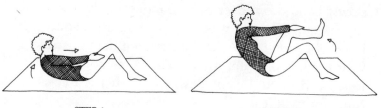

STEP 1   STEP 2

1. Lie on your back, spine pressed against the floor, knees bent. Raise body in a slow rolling motion while you raise your right leg, knee still bent, to chest level. Touch your fingers to your toes, then slowly roll back down. Repeat 15 times each leg.

2. Lie on your back, hands behind your head, knees bent on your chest. Lift your head and shoulders while you extend your legs in the air, being sure to keep your waist pressed firmly on the floor. Slowly lower body to starting position. Repeat 10 times, or more if you can.

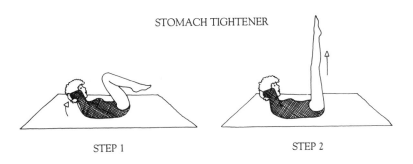

STOMACH TIGHTENER

STEP 1   STEP 2

WAIST WHITTLER

Sit on floor, legs straight and spread a hip's width apart, arms over head with hands clasped. Stretch up high and slowly bend down over right leg, pushing hands out to touch your right toe, if you can. If you bend your knee just slightly, you will take the strain off the underside of your thigh. Come up, stretch, and come down between legs. Bend up and come down over left leg. Repeat 10 times for each leg.

WHOLE BODY STRETCH

This should be the first and last exercise you do to un-wind and stretch out your body. Stand tall, feet a hip's width apart, arms above your head, hands clasped. Stretch up as tall as you can, reaching toward the ceiling with your clasped hands. Slowly roll your body down and bend your knees slightly. Push your clasped hands against your right foot. Stretch up again and come down in between legs, pushing hands on floor. Come up again and stretch, bend over left foot, and push hands against it. Repeat 3 times on each side.

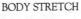

BODY STRETCH

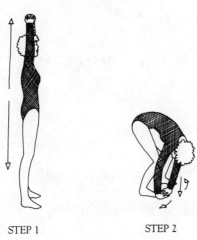

STEP 1   STEP 2

UPPER-ARM SHAPER

If you are not as happy as you used to be wearing short sleeves and bare-armed clothes, this exercise is for you. Stand tall, feet a hip's width apart. Slowly bend over until your body forms a right angle. Let your arms hang down. Bend your arms and press elbows tightly against your body; hold for a count of five. Straighten your arms out in back of you and press upper arms tightly against your body. Hold for a count of five. Let arms drop down and repeat 10 times.

C H A P T E R 11

T I M E S O F
S T R E S S — T I M E S
O F G R O W T H

From the day you first try, as a baby, to reach that in-
triguing, shiny object just beyond your grasp, frustration
and stress are part of your life. As a baby, you cried
when you couldn't have what you wanted. As a child,
you threw temper tantrums. As an adult, frustration
takes on different guises. You feel frustration just as
acutely as you did as a child, but now you can't have a
tantrum. Instead you may internalize your frustration
and become depressed. Some situations in adult life may
be so stressful—a new job, loss of an old one, death of a
loved one, financial pressures—that you experience real
panic. More often, you have human highs and lows, periods of real happiness contrasted with periods of depres-

sion and stress. To feel stress, a friend once said, is the only sure sign of being alive.

The most basic form of stress, common to all human beings and activated whenever your life is actually threatened—or you perceive it to be—is the *fight-or-flight response.* When you feel you are in a life-threatening situation, your hypothalamus sends out signals to increase your supply of epinephrine (adrenaline) and norepinephrine (noradrenaline). Your pituitary gland also activates other hormones, and soon your blood is rich in all kinds of life-protecting chemicals and hormones designed to help you fend off the impending threat. It is these chemicals and hormones that enable you to do "superhuman" things to protect yourself and others in times of acute stress. Your stimulated body chemistry gives you the power to fight back or to flee, whichever is most appropriate for the situation.

Most stressful situations, however, don't call for this kind of basic, primitive body response. Especially in midlife, you are much more likely to feel certain kinds of low-level, but insidious stress and depression. One of the most difficult things about midlife is that, at age forty or thereabouts, you can no longer play "When I grow up" with yourself. Through your teens, your twenties, and thirties, you could safely feel that if you had not gotten the high-level job you dreamed of, or you had not yet been able to afford the big house with a swimming pool, or you could not buy the designer clothes you always fantasized about, you would be able to have all this "later." The later was some vague, fuzzy time in the future. Life still lay in front of you, ready to fulfill your dreams and fantasies any day, any year. But now, at forty, and the beginning of midlife, you are likely to have your first sneaky suspicion that the life you have is all you are going to get. If the big job isn't in the offing by now, or you still don't have the down payment on that bigger house, or your marriage isn't the romantic experience you used to dream about, chances are, you are going to have to do some *rearranging of your expectations.*

This coming to grips with the reality of your life is an important aspect of midlife. Everyone must do it, and sometimes, if your expectations and your reality are very far apart, you go through a period of intense disappointment, frustration, and stress, until you begin to accept your life for what it really is and what it has the realistic chance of becoming. *Finding a new equilibrium* is a delicate business and may take several years, during which time you may feel unhappy and unfulfilled.

This is a perfectly normal experience and, in fact, a very important one. Until you have moved through this period and come out the other end successfully, you cannot get on with the next, happier stage of your life.

Your distress at this time is usually caused because you feel you are not the person you thought you would become. It is true that most of us have to make some basic adjustments as we grow older. We all had dreams of grandeur as youths. These dreams made us grow, but now you need to move beyond the dreams and start enjoying the life you have, while still being able to look forward to many good things in the future. One way you can help yourself get through this period of adjustment is to look at yourself realistically. You are probably selling yourself short.

IDEAL PERSON EXERCISE

Try this exercise and see who you really are. First sit down and make a list of your characteristics. Think positively. Are you intelligent, loyal, faithful, adventuresome, honest? What qualities define you? Now make a second list. What qualities would your ideal person have? Should she be sincere, intelligent, amusing? Compare your two lists. Ellen, a forty-two-year-old woman who tried this exercise, had lists that looked like this.

My Qualities	Ideal Qualities
Smart	Intelligent
Thoughtful	Sincere
Shy	Trustworthy
Pretty	Attractive
Upbeat	Assertive
Sincere	Positive outlook
	Caring of others

Ellen was surprised to see how many qualities appeared on both her lists. She realized that though she had been going through a period of unhappiness and self-depreciation, she was actually very much like her "ideal" person in meaningful ways. When our real qualities match our ideal ones, psychologists say we are *integrated or self-actualized human beings*. Although some of the trappings of your life—clothes, home, income—may fall short of your dreams, your basic human qualities may have developed much as you wanted. Realizing that can improve your self-image and relieve a great deal of midlife stress. In areas where your two lists don't match, there is often a lot you can do to make them jibe.

One basic area of disagreement in Ellen's list was in the area of assertiveness. Ellen admired assertiveness and felt that she was shy and lacking in this quality. If you ask yourself what would happen if you took on the quality you lack, you may find that change is not as forbidding as it might seem. Ellen felt that people, especially her husband, would see her as bossy and unfeminine, if she became more assertive. Once she realized this was what she feared, she was able to test out her fear and see how valid the assumption was. She began speaking up more, asking for what she wanted, and tried to be more outgoing. To her surprise, her husband responded positively. Instead of finding her bossy, he found her more attractive and more stimulating as a person. Being more outgoing helped her enjoy people more, especially in situations where she met new people. For Ellen, this was an important discovery.

Cynthia, another woman who tried this exercise, found that she fell short of her ideal in the area of attractiveness. Cynthia had let her looks fall apart. She had gained weight, had let her hair go unattractively gray, did not enjoy shopping for clothes or taking care of herself. Five years before, her husband had left her for a younger woman whom Cynthia saw as much more attractive. Afraid of being hurt again, Cynthia had decided then and there that she would no longer compete in terms of looks. Finally, realizing that what she had done made her angry with herself, she decided to pull herself together. "It may not win me a man," she said, "but at least it can win back my own self-respect." And it did.

Look at your own list, see where you fall short, and ask yourself what you are afraid of. It may be a fear you have developed only recently, one that is related to aging, but it is just as likely that it is a fear you have had all your life. There is no time like right now for coming to terms with it.

IT CAN'T HAPPEN TO ME

In addition to forcing us to come to grips with the reality of our lives and the stuff of our dreams, midlife throws us another curve. Somewhere around age forty, you probably have your first fleeting, but real, confrontation with the fact that pretty little, young little you can grow old just like everyone else. In the past, you probably looked at women forty and beyond as inhabitants of another world, one you would never enter because you had your youth and you would always have it. If you are lucky enough to have a long life, you won't always have youth. You, too, will become part of the world peopled by "older" types. Accepting your own aging process and dealing with the fact that you are no longer a *young* woman is as important as dealing with the fact that many of the things you dreamed of having and becoming may be lost to you. Until you accept the aging process as something that applies to you, you cannot move on to the next productive stage of your life.

WHAT HELPS

The kinds of stress we have been talking about so far are different from most other stresses that we experience throughout life. Dealing with them is a must for emotional growth. One of the most healing things you can do is to talk with other women your own age and older. You will discover one of two things. Either these women will deny totally that they are feeling what you are feeling—and you can conclude they are deceiving themselves—or you will experience an outpouring of feelings similar to your own. When this happens, really listen to what the other woman is saying, and you will discover that you are not alone. Knowing that almost every other woman your age has felt what you are feeling now can be very comforting. Talk about your mutual feelings and allow them to engulf you for a time. Admitting to them, owning up to your feelings, and experiencing them at their fullest is the only way you can move beyond them. The next step is, indeed, to move beyond them. Do not let yourself become stuck in this readjustment period too long. Begin to focus on what lies ahead of you. The new energy, new beginnings, and excitement of this part of your life can be as stimulating as the excitement you felt at the end of your teens when you stood on the brink of adulthood.

There are many new, positive things to look forward to. Here is a list of some; you can add many of your own.

THE COMMON, EVERYDAY STRESSES

So far, we have talked about the special stresses of midlife, but in addition, there are other stresses that we all share, no matter what our age. From time to time, there will be stress over job or family problems, over not hav-

THINGS YOU CAN LOOK FORWARD TO NOW

The pleasure of children—your children's children—without the responsibility of raising them

A freer and more interesting sex life, as you pass through the menopause and don't have to worry about an unwanted pregnancy

More private time of your own

The chance to actually do some of the things you only used to dream about—travel, get a job, get a better job, take a course, write

The entire second half of your life—since life expectancy, especially for women, is increasing

Establishing "adult" ties with your children

Improving your relationship with your husband now that most of the stresses of child raising are over

Concentrating more on *your* wants and needs

Having the time to improve your looks

ing the time you need to accomplish what you want, of having to wait in line too long, of simply having a bad day. Unlike the special stresses of midlife, these are the kinds of stress you can never expect will disappear completely. These are the stresses you must learn to cope with.

WHY SHOULD YOU LEARN TO COPE?

If you are taking the trouble to read this book, you are interested in the way you look. Try to catch a glimpse of yourself when you feel tense or stressed. You are not at your best, are you? You look pinched, you are probably frowning, or at least not looking pleasant. Stress is a beauty spoiler, and this is one good reason to learn to deal constructively with it. More important, it is also a health spoiler. Prolonged stress is often associated with disease. Researchers are not sure what the relationship between stress and disease is, but they know that the two are closely related. Recent research indicates that when we are under stress for long periods of time, and our bodies are bathed in stress-related chemicals, our immune system breaks down and we succumb to diseases that we would ordinarily be able to resist. Whatever the relationship, it is important to learn to deal with stress so that it does not make you sick.

Sometimes your own attitude can be causing you more stress than necessary. To find out if this is true for you, ask yourself these questions.

What are my real life goals? Am I striving for them or something I only think I want?

Am I pursuing my own goals or someone else's?

Am I maintaining healthy attitudes about dealing with stress, or am I letting stress get the best of me?

Do I allow myself enough private time?

Am I as aware of the good things about myself as I should be?

Do I give myself enough opportunity to get away from it all—do I plan for real vacations away from my normal routine a couple of times a year?

WHAT HELPS

The right answers to the questions above can help a great deal. Do you really know what your life goals are? Have you actually thought about them recently? If you are pressing madly on in a job, because ten years ago job success was the most important thing in your life, is it still so important? After working and succeeding for many years, perhaps now what you would really like best is to slow down and relax a bit. Unless you examine your present goals, you may be working for goals you have outgrown.

Are your goals your own? Or are they goals your family imposed on you? If your parents wanted you to make a good marriage and that is what you did, is that still central to your life? Would you like to pursue something *you* want now—like a job, perhaps for the first time? Or perhaps you married the "right" man according to your parent's choice, but it has been a less than ideal marriage for you. Perhaps now is the time to reexamine the marriage and see if you still want to stay in it.

If you are in a period of stress, how healthy are your attitudes? Do you firmly believe the stress will pass? Or are you succumbing to constant panic? If you are not handling the stress well, perhaps you could get professional help. A therapist may be able to make this temporary period easier for you to live through.

One of the most important gifts you can give yourself

is private time. Some time alone to renew and refresh ourselves is something we all need. It may be an hour in the morning when you read the paper in bed with no interruptions. It may be a forty-five-minute solitary walk to work to give you time to refuel for the day. It could be an hour before bedtime to do exactly what you want, with no interruptions. Whenever it is, it is vitally important that you schedule some private time for yourself.

Do you sell yourself short? Don't. This practice can be energy killing, beauty spoiling, life threatening. Try the Ideal Person Exercise mentioned earlier in this chapter and keep working on yourself until you become a more self-content person.

No matter how good your life may be, it has some sort of routine, and routines become boring after a while. The only way to break out is to take a vacation. It does not have to cost a lot of money or involve going far away, but it must involve changing your routine. No matter who you are or what you do on a daily basis, you need regular change. One woman who seemed to have the perfect life—a good job, a beautiful apartment in the city, and a lovely house in the country—expressed it this way: "People think I'm crazy and indulgent when I insist we take a vacation every fall. They can't understand why having a summer house isn't a summer-long vacation. But driving to that house every weekend and entertaining friends almost every week becomes as much of a routine as going to a dreary job day after day. You need a change to feel refreshed, so I insist on getting away."

You can often exercise your way through temporary stress. Trite as it may seem, *activity is one of the best relaxers.*

Test out this idea if you don't believe it. The next time you feel especially stressed or frustrated or depressed, take a good, long walk. Get up some speed so you are moving along at a good pace. Or try a swim, a fast game of tennis, or go jogging. After an hour of vigorous physical activity, you will feel better. Exercise, like stress, releases certain chemicals into your bloodstream. The chemical release associated with stress is negative, but exercise causes a positive chemical release. These chemicals account for the "high" athletes often get when they are in the midst of vigorous activity. You won't experience this "high" unless you exercise vigorously, so don't settle for a ten-minute walk and expect to feel better. Get out and get your body moving.

Face what is making you tense and see if there is anything you can do about it. If you feel tense and anxious because you hate your job or because you are having continuous fights with your husband, face facts and see if you can change any aspects of the situation. Often you can. Perhaps you can change enough things about your job to remove a big portion of the stress. If, for example, you continually feel you have too much work to do, you could talk it over with your supervisor and see if there isn't some way you can unload a portion of your work. If you are fighting with your husband more than usual, take yourselves out to dinner one night when you are both in a good mood and discuss the matter. See if the two of you together can figure out why you have been battling so much and determine what can be done about it. Even if your marriage is falling apart, it might be better to face this and end the marriage rather than prolonging the unhappiness.

Accept the fact that life is never stress-free and that,

many times, you will simply outlive the stressful situation. If you have lost your job or your husband has lost his, keep reminding yourself that as stressful as the present undoubtedly is, this too shall pass; there are better times ahead. This will help you survive the present. If you are distressed over a problem your grown child is having, remember that your child is an adult now, and he or she must solve his or her own problems. You are no longer the appropriate problem solver. If you have given your children emotionally healthy childhoods, they will be able to solve their problems just as you have solved yours.

Remember that life is a series of highs and lows, and you can enjoy the highs in contrast to the lows. A life of only highs would be boring and a life of all lows unendurable. By living through the lows, we are able to savor the triumphs of the highs.

Remember that it is because of the periods of stress we live through that we grow. Without stress—and the realization that you can cope with whatever life has in store for you—you would stop growing. As you cope, you grow. Did you ever hear of anyone becoming a better person because she experienced so much happiness?

INSTANT DE-STRESSING EXERCISING

When you are feeling tense, try this quick-relaxation exercise and feel better instantly.

Stand straight, with your feet about a hip's width apart, knees slightly bent, arms back slightly. Now lean over. Hang your head and arms down and just let your body hang loose for a few seconds. Now curl back up and repeat the movement three or four times.

ACTION CHECKLIST FOR CONTROLLING STRESS

• Reappraise your youthful expectations to bring them into sync with midlife realities.

• Work on becoming a more self-content human being.

• Accept the fact that you, like the rest of the world, are growing older.

• Focus on the good things that you have to look forward to for the next half of your life.

• Schedule private time to refresh yourself.

• Use exercise to relax.

• Accept the fact that stress is a life force. It constantly reappears in everyone's life and it can be handled.

LIVING WITH STRESS

WHAT THE EXPERTS SAY

Dr. Mary Boulton, director of the Gotham Institute of Transactional Analysis, has been helping people cope with stress for years. She has a large private practice in New York City where she also runs group-therapy sessions and weekend seminars for people of all ages. Her warm and caring attitude has made her beloved by her patients, many of whom keep up with her years after their therapy is finished. Here is her approach to coping with midlife stress.

Is the experience of getting older a stressful one?

It can be, if you choose to make it one. We are all growing older constantly; you can decide whether this experience is awful or exciting. It's really up to you. I look at ageism just as I do sexism. They are both something we have to combat.

Why do some people grow older gracefully and others become bitter?

Aging is just another of life's many experiences and, as with any experience, it's your attitude toward it that determines the outcome. If you view turning forty as the beginning of the end, it will be. If you view it as an exciting new milestone in your life, then that's exactly what it will be. We have it within our power to control so many aspects of our lives, if we just do it. It's true that our culture doesn't make it easy for us to age gracefully. In some cultures, such as the Chinese, age is revered. Older people are honored for their wisdom. We tend to treat older people as we do single people. If you're not young, you don't belong. If you're not part of a couple, you don't belong. Both attitudes are silly.

Why is menopause so stressful for so many women?

The stress comes primarily from ignorance. We confuse menopause with loss of sexual desire and with desirability itself. It's important to know that sexual desire and performance continue into your seventies and eighties. I had a sixty-one-year-old patient who had gone back to college to get her degree. She came to see me the day after she learned she'd passed her exams and earned her degree at last. I asked her what she did to celebrate and she said she went home and made love with her husband. It's important to remember that desire and the ability to act on it go on and on. A woman can have an orgasm without her partner's penis entering her vagina, so even if aging has made penetration impossible, sex is still very possible. Women have so little information about what happens to their bodies as they age; this lack of information is what causes much of the stress at midlife.

How can you handle the stress and depression of midlife when you do experience it?

Activity is a great stress reliever. It can be the activity of exercise or of some new interest. Colleges and universities all across the country are realizing how valuable education later in life can be. Many colleges now offer credit for life experiences to make it easier for midlife men and women to go back to school. Women should take advantage of this opportunity. It can help them find new value in their lives.

Also, as a society, we are reexamining our ideas of success. We are much more flexible when we define success. A job or career that causes great stress can be dropped in favor of something we like to do more. We are redefining success to encompass fulfillment and contentment. Success doesn't always have to be economic or even professional—success can be doing what gives you pleasure and rewards you personally. We no longer expect everyone to get ahead monolithically. To be considered a success, you don't have to work your way up the corporate ladder if you find much more satisfaction in a hands-on job. This is a big and welcome change.

C H A P T E R 12

Y O U R

Q U E S T I O N S

A N S W E R E D

Every life stage presents us with dilemmas, and midlife is no exception. Here are some of the most commonly asked questions and their no-nonsense answers.

B E A U T Y

I'm beginning to see a lot of very fine wrinkles on my cheeks and around my eyes. I'm a heavy smoker. Could this have anything to do with the wrinkling?

No one knows for certain, but the evidence is beginning to build that smoking, especially heavy smoking, does produce these fine wrinkles. Researchers are not quite sure why or what the mechanism is, but since these fine wrinkles—which, incidentally, deepen as you age—so often are associated with heavy smok-

ing, it seems logical to assume a connection. The evidence against smoking from both a beauty and health standpoint is overwhelming. Anyone who is really interested in staying healthy and looking good should stop smoking.

The ends of my hair are very dry and splitting badly. I've never had this problem before, but since I've started using a curling iron frequently I've become aware of lots of split ends. Is the curling iron the cause?

The curling iron is definitely the problem if you have not had trouble with split ends before. Your hair is probably not as oily now as it once was, and the curling iron dries it out even more, especially the ends. You can continue to use your curling iron, but you should use a conditioner on your hair regularly. Try using one every other time you shampoo, and you should see improvement. In the meantime, have your ends trimmed regularly until you get rid of all the dry split portions of hair.

My blusher collects on the dry, flaky part of my cheeks and looks terrible, yet I don't want to give up wearing it. What can I do?

If you are not already using one, switch to a cream blusher. It will absorb into your skin more and the dry-skin flakes won't be so noticeable. Be certain, also, to use a good moisturizer in this area, and remember to use a sloughing product regularly to remove those dead-skin flakes. In your case, a buffing puff used to wash your face a couple of times a week would probably help considerably. You might also experiment with a grainy scrub cleanser. Use whichever works best for you.

I'd like to try a new hairstyle with bangs but I don't know whether bangs are becoming at my age. I'm forty-five.

Bangs can be becoming at any age. They can make you look youthful and fresh. They do, however, draw attention to eyes, so if you're going to wear bangs, your eyes should be in good shape. If you have a lot of little lines, sags, or puffs, bangs may not be a good idea.

My lipstick bleeds terribly at my lip line, making it look smeary. I can't give up lipstick, yet I hate this look. What can I do?

Try a lip pencil, one with a hard consistency in a tawny color. Apply your lipstick just inside the line of the pencil. This will help considerably. Also, experiment with different lipsticks. Avoid the creamiest types; they bleed most. There are also a couple of products on the market designed for this problem. One is a cream applied under lipstick that seems to work well for some women. The idea is that the cream moisturizes and temporarily plumps out and fills in the tiny lines that cause lipstick to bleed. Another product that works especially well, but that is hard to find in some parts of the country, is a liquid fixative that you apply over lip color. It dries quickly and forms a protective covering. If you just use it around your lip line, it is very effective.

I must wear glasses to read, and the magnifying lens magnifies the lines around my eyes. What can I do?

Try a tinted lens. Pick a soft brown or rose tint, nothing too dark; just a suggestion of color will help. A tinted lens acts like eye makeup and makes the magnifying effect less noticeable.

I am beginning to notice unattractive brown spots on the backs of my hands. They make me feel old. What can I do about them?

There are several creams on the market that fade these pigmented spots, but you must use them for a long time before you notice results, and you must continue to use them or sun exposure will cause the spots to return. A better idea, if you don't have a lot of spots, is to have your dermatologist remove them. It is a simple procedure and usually not expensive. You may have a very faint white "scar" as a result, but this is barely noticeable and far preferable to the brown spot, which will probably get larger and darker as time goes by.

Though I have quite a good figure, my upper arms are getting flabby and I don't like the way they look in sleeveless or short-sleeved clothes. What can I do?

Try this quick exercise. Hold your arms out in front of you, elbows bent, hands clasped together. Clasp your hands as tightly as you can for a count of five. Repeat a half dozen times a day.

I see little fat dimples on the backs of my legs. I guess this is what many women call cellulite. What can I do about it?

Cellulite is plain ordinary fat. Some people seem to have more of this dimpling problem than others. To get rid of the dimples, you must get rid of the fat. Unfortunately, this condition frequently occurs in the areas that are hardest to reduce; and, often, even though you have lost the amount of weight you want, the dimpled skin remains. The only solution is to lose more weight, which in many cases is not desirable. You may have to put up with some cellulite, although if you are at a good weight, you should be able to get rid of most of it. Don't be fooled by diets or gadgets that promise to remove cellulite. None really work. Overall weight loss is the only solution. No special foods or combination of foods or products will get rid of the problem magically.

I had cosmetic surgery on my eyelids about eight years ago and I feel they need to be done again. Is this possible?

Usually it is possible to have eyelids lifted a second time with great success. There are a few instances when it is not a good idea, but only your plastic surgeon can determine if there would be problems in your case.

I have heard people talk about acupuncture face lifts. What are they, and do they work?

There are indeed some acupuncturists who are using this ancient method to improve facial contours. One doctor described an acupuncture face lift as something between a facial and a surgical lift. Many women feel that they do notice improvement, but the improvement, if there is any, is temporary. You have to return for additional lifts. An acupuncture lift is no substitute for a surgical lift, which produces permanent and predictable results.

DIET/FITNESS

I exercise for ten minutes every night before I go to bed. Is this helping to keep me fit?

Ten minutes of exercise, even if it is done daily, is useless as far as overall fitness is concerned. If you are doing it to shape up a particular area, such as your stomach muscles, ten minutes of sit-ups will certainly firm your stomach, but they will do nothing for overall fitness. You need to do aerobic exercise—exercise that increases your heart rate—for at least twenty to thirty minutes three to four times a week to do anything for fitness.

I walk to work every day, but I have to stop at lights. Does this exercise help keep me fit?

As good as walking to work is for you in other ways, if you must stop and start often, walking does not produce aerobic benefits. To achieve aerobic benefits, you must sustain your in-creased heartbeat for at least twenty minutes. In the time you are waiting for a red light to turn green, your heartbeat slows down. See if you can't find some other place to walk where you can go for twenty minutes without having to stop. If time is a problem, you would be wiser to take the bus or drive to work and do your walking where you can walk nonstop.

I play tennis doubles every weekend. Is this keeping me fit?

Tennis is fun, and playing certainly burns up calories, but it is a stop-and-start activity and produces no aerobic benefits. It is a wonderful de-stressing exercise, however, because it absorbs you, gets you away from your problems, and gets you out with people.

I absolutely hate to exercise. Can I be fit without it?

Although many people do live their lives without it, we know that keeping fit with exercise dramatically increases your chances of good health and longevity. Fitness is a relative thing and is influenced by many things. It is impossible to determine whether you are "fit" for your age without an exercise stress test that checks how your body responds to increased activity. You would also have to take a flexibility test to see how much flexi-bility you have lost. Only then could you judge how "fit" you are for your age. It is safe to say that if you continue avoiding exercise, you will pay for it in reduced flexibility and energy as you grow older. What degenerative diseases you might develop as a result of inactivity would depend on your particular heredity and susceptibility.

Is it possible to be fit and overweight?

Yes, you can be fit and slightly overweight, but if you are greatly overweight, your excess weight would prevent you from getting the kind of aerobic exercise that keeps you fit. Also, if you are truly fit, you will probably be burning off enough excess calories to keep you trim. Obesity and fitness rarely go hand in hand.

HEALTH

I'm forty-five and I have been having very heavy periods. My last one went on for two weeks. What is happening, and is it serious?

As you age, it is not uncommon to have heavy, irregular periods. Your body is probably being bombarded with estrogen, causing your uterine lining to build up more than usual. When you do have a period, this thick lining is shed for a considerable amount of time. At this age, long periods are usually not a sign of anything serious, but they should not be ignored. Anything over seven or eight days should be reported to your doctor. He or she may want you to have a dilation and curettage to be certain everything is normal. Uterine cysts can sometimes cause excessive bleeding and may require medical attention, or you could have a precancerous condition that should be taken care of before it becomes serious.

I am still menstruating and I have hot flashes. Is this possible?

It is indeed. Once you pass forty, your hormone flow is not so smooth and regular as it once was. You may have months when your ovaries are producing large amounts of estrogen and months when they produce less. During times of decreased estrogen production, you may experience hot flashes. They will usually disappear when your ovaries produce more estrogen. Once you have stopped menstruating altogether, the hot flashes will probably be persistent for a while before they stop completely.

My breasts are swollen and sore for months on end. Is this normal? What causes it?

This commonly happens at midlife. Your ovaries are beginning to run down and your estrogen production is erratic. Your body is producing certain hormones that are intended to stimulate your ovaries to produce more estrogen. When your ovaries do secrete more estrogen, your breasts may become very tender and swollen. You may go for months with high levels of estrogen in your bloodstream, causing you to have sore, engorged breasts. The problem usually vanishes as you actually go through menopause. If your breasts are excessively painful, you should see your doctor.

My breasts have suddenly become lumpy and what my doctor calls cystic. Why is this happening now?

Once again, increased and erratic estrogen production is probably the cause. Some women respond to increased estrogen production by producing small cysts in their breasts. The cysts are harmless, but when they appear suddenly, many women become fearful and think they are developing breast cancer. You should stay in close contact with your gynecologist during this time to be certain there are no problems. Most women have difficulty knowing when a lump is a harmless cyst and what may mean trouble. Checking with your doctor every four to six months will ease your mind. The cystic condition often disappears after menopause.

Another cause of cystic breasts in women of all ages is apparently caffeine. Most women can drink tea or coffee and colas with no ill effects, but in others, the caffeine produces a cystic condition. In this case, you must give up any beverage with caffeine in it—namely tea, coffee, and cola drinks—and any over-the-counter medication that contains caffeine (many do—check the labels of anything you take regularly). Many women with cystic breasts find giving up caffeine reduces their problems measurably. You cannot expect to see positive results for six months or so, and should be prepared to have slight caffeine withdrawal symptoms—the most troublesome is a severe headache. All symptoms of withdrawal usually vanish within two weeks.

I have been divorced for five years and have not had sex. Now, at fifty, I've met a man I'm in love with and I want to have sex, but I'm afraid I will find it painful. What can I do?

This is a delicate problem. Being fearful will only make it worse. It is best to see your gynecologist and have him or her prescribe an estrogen cream to use vaginally for a while. In addition, you should buy a surgical lubricating jelly to use just before sex. If all this sounds rather unromantic to you, remember that many women and men do not consider a diaphragm or a condom romantic and you, at least, will not have to worry about either *of these. You can apply the lubricant just before sex and your lover need be none the wiser. As you become more secure with each other, perhaps you can incorporate applying the lubricant into your lovemaking. Many couples do and find that it adds pleasure to the sex act. It is no different from having your partner insert your diaphragm or making inserting it part of the lovemaking act.*

CHAPTER 21

WHAT IS IT REALLY LIKE

. . .

NOT TO BE A YOUNG WOMAN ANY LONGER?

You can pass forty and still feel and look like a young woman, but sometime shortly after passing this milestone age, the thought crosses your mind, "I'm not young anymore." One woman put it this way: "I passed forty and thought nothing of it, and never gave age any thought for several years. Then, at forty-four, it suddenly occurred to me, 'My God, I'm soon going to be closer to fifty than forty.' I panicked." Another woman said, "I used to think men had it made and I was bitter. I was forty-five and my husband was fifty-one and he was still considered 'young' and handsome. I felt over the hill. Then suddenly, he lost his job and started looking for a new one. After six months of desperately hard work, he began to realize that at fifty-one, he was 'too old' for many of the jobs he'd been interviewing for. I stood by, powerless to help, and felt terrible for him. I'll never again feel one-down to a man. They have their troubles, too."

One friend described her feelings this way: "All through my twenties and thirties, I felt young and privileged. I saw my older friends and I thought, 'It's not going to happen to me, I'm young and I'll stay that way.' I tried to think of middle age as being so far down the road it wasn't even a concern. Today, I'm forty-four and it *has* happened to me—and so fast. I can't believe I'm this age." Another woman has what seems to be the most sensible approach. "I stopped thinking of myself as an 'age' years ago. What's the point? When you're sixteen, you don't spend all your time thinking about the experience of being a teen-ager. When you're twenty or thirty, you don't fixate on being twenty or thirty, you just live your life. That's what you have to do at forty or fifty or sixty—live your life to the best of your ability. I've grown to believe that every stage of life has its advantages and disadvantages. When I look back over my life, I wouldn't want to be twenty-five again. Getting smart was too hard. I would never want to be that naïve and that vulnerable and that stupid again!"

It is true, every age does have its advantages; and midlife has a lot of them. For the first time, many women find themselves really free—free of family responsibilities, sometimes even economic responsibilities to children or others. For some, this freedom can be frightening, but it need not be. With life expectancy growing, you have another forty years before you, and it can indeed be the best forty years. Most elderly people are not unhappy; in fact, research shows that many of them feel they have an easier time and fewer cares than they had in adolescence and in their twenties and thirties when they were competing so hard to get ahead financially and professionally.

A psychologist recently told a reassuring story. She has a friend, a former patient, who was just celebrating her seventy-eighth birthday. The woman said she was happier and more fulfilled now than she had ever been in her life. Her relationship with her children was excellent, she volunteered time three days a week to work with disturbed children, and the rest of the time she puttered around her house and worked in her garden. "I have the ideal life," she said. "When I think back on how tumultuous my youth was, how hard I worked to raise my children, and how much I worried about being middle-aged, I realize how good things are today."

If we, like this woman, can see the years ahead as full and rewarding, midlife holds no terrors. It also has something else to offer. Most of us are freer now than we have ever been before. We cannot afford to sit back and be complacent or unconcerned. Men, with their power, status, and influence, are missing something we can supply. In this age of up-and-down inflation and interest rates, of unemployment, uncertain economics, and nuclear terror, women remain the ones who have been socialized to be the caretakers, the nurturers. In our early years, many of us were busy caring for and nurturing our families, but now, at forty and more, we can turn our attention to society as a whole. It is women who can add humane values to business and politics—but we cannot do it by sitting back and feeling sorry for ourselves as middle-aged frumps or over-the-hill citizens. Midlife women are our most underused natural asset, and it is time we realized it. It is time we got out and got involved with something besides our own little world. It's time we started working to make things better for all of us. Women may never have quite the same clout in some areas as men, but that may be a hidden blessing. While males are brought up to be aggressive and assertive, to be the big risk-takers, women are still being brought up to be the keepers of true humanity. At midlife, a good many of us come into our own with a long stretch of relatively carefree time in front of us. We must be the ones who work to spread that humanity. Like the torch bearers at the Olympics, women are the torch bearers of our society. There is no time like midlife to take up that torch and start running with it.

I N D E X